DEAN CLOSE SCHOOL

LIBRARY

This book must be returned by the latest date stamped below

WILLIAM HARVEY

AND THE

CIRCULATION OF THE BLOOD

History of Science Library

Editor: MICHAEL A. HOSKIN
Lecturer in the History of Science, Cambridge University

THE ENGLISH PARACELSIANS
Allen G. Debus
Professor of the History of Science, University of Chicago

WILLIAM HERSCHEL AND THE CONSTRUCTION OF THE HEAVENS
M. A. Hoskin
Lecturer in the History of Science, Cambridge University

A HISTORY OF THE THEORIES OF RAIN
W. E. Knowles Middleton

THE ORIGINS OF CHEMISTRY
R. P. Multhauf
Director of the Museum of History and Technology at the Smithsonian Institution

THEORIES OF LIGHT FROM DESCARTES TO NEWTON
A. I. Sabra
Reader in the History of the Classical Tradition, The Warburg Institute

MEDICINE IN MEDIEVAL ENGLAND
C. H. Talbot
Research Fellow at the Wellcome Institute of the History of Medicine, London

THE EARTH IN DECAY
A HISTORY OF BRITISH GEOMORPHOLOGY, 1578–1878
G. L. Davies
Lecturer in the Department of Geography, Trinity College, University of Dublin

THE CONFLICT BETWEEN ATOMISM AND CONSERVATION THEORY 1644–1860
W. L. Scott
Professorial Lecturer, School of Business Administration and Department of Mathematics and Science, American University

THE ROAD TO MEDICAL ENLIGHTENMENT 1650–1695
L. S. King
Professorial Lecturer in the History of Medicine, University of Chicago

THE SCIENTIFIC ORIGINS OF NATIONAL SOCIALISM:
SOCIAL DARWINISM IN ERNST HAECKEL AND THE GERMAN MONIST LEAGUE
Daniel Gasman
Assistant Professor of History, John Jay College, The City University of New York

History of Science Library: Primary Sources

VEGETABLE STATICKS
Stephen Hales
Foreword by M. A. Hoskin
Lecturer in the History of Science, Cambridge University

SCIENCE AND EDUCATION IN THE SEVENTEENTH CENTURY
THE WEBSTER-WARD DEBATE
Allen G. Debus
Professor of the History of Science, University of Chicago

FUNDAMENTA MEDICINAE
Friedrich Hoffmann
Translated and introduced by L. S. King
Professorial Lecturer in the History of Medicine, University of Chicago

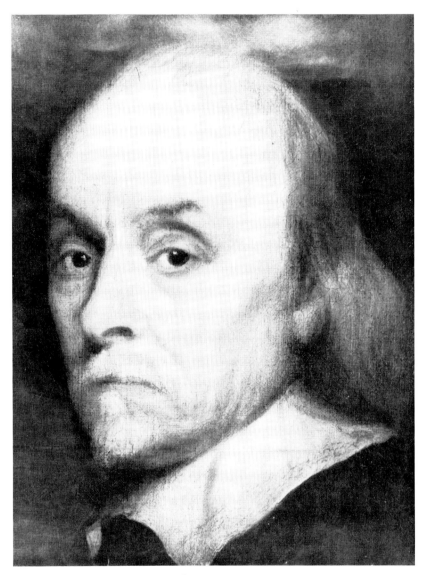

William Harvey

WILLIAM HARVEY

AND THE
CIRCULATION OF
THE BLOOD

GWENETH WHITTERIDGE

M.A., D. Phil., F.S.A.

Lecturer in the History of Medicine
University of Edinburgh

MACDONALD · LONDON
AND
AMERICAN ELSEVIER INC.: NEW YORK

For
D. W.

© Gweneth Whitteridge 1971
First published 1971
Sole distributors for the United States and Dependencies
American Elsevier Publishing Company, Inc.
52 Vanderbilt Avenue
New York, N.Y. 10017

Sole distributors for the British Isles and Commonwealth
Macdonald & Co. (Publishers) Ltd
49–50 Poland Street
London W1A 2LG

All remaining areas
Elsevier Publishing Company
P.O. Box 211
Jan van Galenstraat 335
Amsterdam
The Netherlands

Library of Congress Catalog Card Number 70–114271
Standard Book Numbers
British SBN 356 02699 x
American SBN 444 19663 3

Printed in Great Britain by Hazell Watson & Viney Ltd
Aylesbury, Bucks

Acknowledgements

IN the writing of this book I have acquired many debts which I acknowledge with gratitude. I should like to thank my own college, Lady Margaret Hall, Oxford, for making me its Suzette Taylor Research Fellow and thus enabling me to work in the archives of the University and City of Padua and in those of the Ecole de Médicine in Paris. In Padua, I should like particularly to thank the University's archivist, Dotoressa Lucia Rossetti, and the staff of the Archivio di Stato. In Paris, my thanks go to Mademoiselle Paule Dumaître and the other librarians of the Bibliothèque de l'Ecole de Médicine.

I owe a very deep debt of gratitude to the Librarian and the the the staff of the University Library of Edinburgh, especially to Mr R. J. F. Carnon. I have worked from the first editions of all Harvey's writings, both Latin and English, owned by the University Library, as well as from its copies, usually first editions, of the works of his predecessors and contemporaries. I should also like to thank the Scottish Carnegie Trust for their support during part of the time that this book was being written.

I should like to thank the Royal College of Physicians of London for their permission to reproduce the portrait of Harvey, and the librarian, Mr Payne, for answering many questions.

I am grateful to Dr Michael Hoskin and to Mrs Rowy Mitchison for reading the typescript of this book and for making helpful suggestions and comments.

EDINBURGH 1969   G. W.

Contents

                                                                   vii

Plates

Preface

THE reader of this book will find in it the history of a discovery, not an account of a theory of discovery. Beginning from Harvey's university studies, I have tried to find out by what steps he came to the realisation that the blood circulated throughout the whole body. Because I believe that Harvey falls into the category of the great scientist who is not conscious of any philosophical method underlying his actions, yet by these actions advances knowledge, I have tried to pay attention to what he did. For Harvey, the primary necessity underlying all his actions is personal observation. On this there is constant insistence in all his work. In the Second Letter to Riolan, he explains how he has endeavoured to show the circulation

> by my observations and experiments, and not to demonstrate by causes and probable principles, but to confirm it by sense and experience, as by a powerful authority, according to the rule of the anatomists (p. 182).

The authority of the book of Nature outweighs the opinions of all the scholars. Phenomena which are manifest to the senses are totally indifferent to any man's opinion concerning them, 'for there is nothing more ancient than Nature or of greater authority' (p. 166). So the pores in the septum, the fuliginous vapours, the doctrine of the spirits, all these hypothetical deductions from ancient systems, Harvey first clears from his mind and begins to observe what actually goes on in the body. There can be little doubt that Harvey's great admiration for Aristotle rests primarily on Aristotle's capacity for patient observation of Nature. Whatever Harvey may say in his *De generatione* about 'the method I use in searching into things', it is plain that his own achievement was brought about simply by this same means of patient and repeated observation. It is characteristic of Harvey, that this, the very basis of his creed he finds in Aristotle. In *De generatione*, having quoted from the *Metaphysics* to the effect that all knowledge comes to man through the senses and experience, he concludes that by this Aristotle

> clearly shows that no man can be truly called prudent or knowledgeable who does not by his own experience (attained by manifold remembrances, frequent perception by his senses and diligent observation) understand that a thing is so. For without all this, we only surmise or believe; and such a knowledge is to be deemed other men's rather than our own. Wherefore fond and erroneous is that method of seeking truth in use in our own times, in which very many enquire diligently not what things are, but what they are said to be by others; and having inferred a universal conclusion from particular premisses and thence falsely deduced an analogue, do they transmit to us many verisimilitudes for truth itself. . . . For whosoever they be that read the words of authors and do not by the aid of their own senses abstract true representation of the things comprehended in the author's words, they do not conceive in their own minds true ideas but deceitful idols and empty phantasms. And by this means they frame to themselves but shadows and chimaeras, and all their theory or contemplation, which nevertheless they count knowledge, representes nothing but waking men's dreams and sick men's frenzies (p. Blv).

Harvey does not use the Aristotelian method of argument from syllogisms, though of course he knows both of induction and deduction. He does not fly back from his observations to first principles; he seeks only the immediate and efficient cause of the phenomenon. When he had over the years assembled his observations on the movement of the heart and blood, it was the careful consideration of these observations which led him to formulate his hypothesis that the blood circulated throughout the whole body as being the only possible means of accounting for these observations. In this process of formulating the hypothesis, there entered the spark of creative intuition which is not as yet amenable to philosophical analysis. But Harvey knew that only those things which can be proved by anatomical dissection and ocular testimony rest on sure foundations. Observation provides the rock on which foundations can be built; scholastic deductions are but shifting sands. These views occur again and again in all his writings from the

Anatomical Lectures to *De generatione*. His actions based on the observation of Nature laid the foundations for the whole of physiology and showed the way for all future scientific discovery.

> Let us then blush, in this so ample and so wonderful field of Nature, where the rewards are ever greater than the promises, to credit other men's words, and thence coin uncertain problems, to spin out thorny and captious questions. Nature herself must be our adviser; the path she chalks must be our walk; for so while we confer with our own eyes and take our rise from meaner things to higher, we shall at length be received into her inmost secrets (*De generatione*, Preface, p. B2).

The Formation

NOTE ON THE PASSAGES TRANSLATED IN THE TEXT

The quotations from *De motu cordis*, the Letters to Riolan and *De generatione* are taken from the first English translations of 1653, corrected when necessary from the first Latin editions. Quotations from Harvey's other writings are my own translations direct from the Latin texts. The translations of all the other works quoted have been made from the Latin editions cited in the Bibliography or references or both.

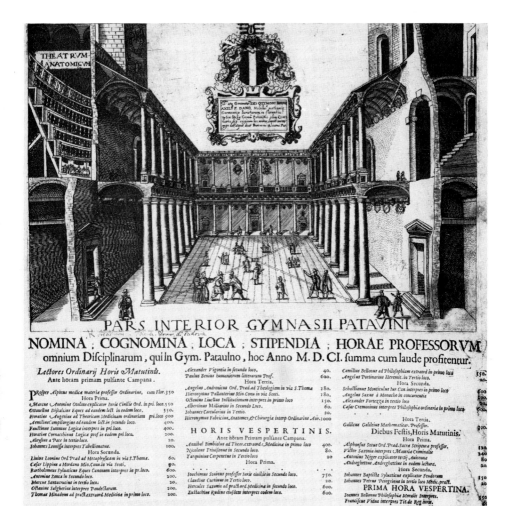

I The official list of professors in the University of Padua 1601

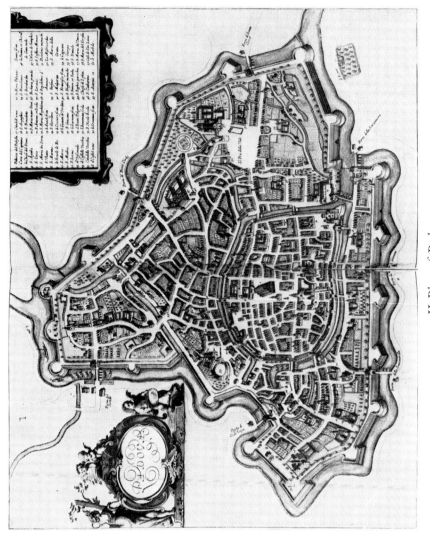

II Plan of Padua

Chapter One

Medical Studies: Cambridge and Padua

IT smacks of the commonplace to say that a man carries through life some vestiges of his early training and education. If his own aptitudes coincide with the interests of those who taught him, particularly during the formative years of his university education, it is likely that his whole intellectual development will be coloured by this teaching and that his maturity will be the fullest working out from the general principles and habits of thought and work learned at this time. Though in many instances this may not be true, in Harvey's case there is no doubt that he carried with him throughout his life the stamp of the University of Padua. There his own interest in natural history was developed into a detailed study of human and comparative anatomy and all that went with it; his powers of observation were fostered and encouraged; his curiosity was sharpened, as he recognised this curiosity as part of the more general enquiry into the secrets of the natural world, an enquiry in which more than one of those who taught him were engaged. There also he found a philosophical approach to learning which fitted his own personality, the rational, unemotional attitude of the Aristotelian. By his discovery of the circulation of the blood Harvey put the keystone to the building which the Paduan anatomists had been raising from the time of Vesalius onwards. But his Aristotelianism made him conservative and perhaps, in some respects, by the end of his life, 'old-fashioned'. He disliked alchemy and undervalued the work of the alchemists, little realising that before the end of the seventeenth century this same alchemy, freed from its mystical, esoteric trappings, would become the science of chemistry. By the middle of the century, though still capable of experimental innovations in his own field, he was not looking forward in any general sense to the developments of the future. His achievement lay in the fact that he had exploited to the full the methods and habits of thought which he had learnt at the university and had gone far beyond them. He had shown that mere observation was not enough; that observation had to be followed by the formulation of an hypothesis, and the validity of this hypothesis tested by experiments expressly designed for that purpose, and that the process had to be repeated over and over again until there was no room for doubt that the true explanation had been found. Whereas, before his time, the question why such or such a phenomenon should occur had not infrequently been asked and had been answered with a multiplicity of false reasons, Harvey saw that in this method of approach there was no way to advance knowledge. From the question *why*, he turned to the question *how*, and in this lies the greatness of his achievement. By observation, by hypothesis and by experiment he answered completely and for all time the question of how the blood moves in the body. The difficulties which lay in the way of his achievement are hard for us to realise, brought up as we are to accept the circulation of the blood as a piece of common knowledge and to take for granted the view that every advance in scientific knowledge proceeds from observation by way of hypothesis and experiment, repeated again and again, until such time as some measure of certainty is reached. For the seventeenth century not only was the concept of the circulation an unheard of novelty, but the method by which it was discovered was equally novel. It was Harvey's example and his achievement which link him directly with his younger friends and pupils, the founders of the Royal Society. He did not pass on to them any philosophical theorising, for in this he did not indulge, but rather the example of a method in action by which results had been achieved.

★   ★   ★

On 31 May 1593, when he was just over fifteen years of age, Harvey matriculated as an ordinary student of Gonville and Caius College, Cambridge. In a university in which at this date medical education on the whole was poor, this college provided the best that could be had. Its second founder and benefactor, John Caius, had completed his own medical career at Padua, where he had been a pupil of Giovanni da Monte and a friend of Vesalius. Realising the basic importance of anatomy for the study of medicine, Caius began to attend dissections in the hall of the Barber-Surgeons' Company in London, shortly after his return to England in 1544 or 1545. A little later he was teaching anatomy there himself, and continued to do so for the next twenty years. Meantime, in 1547, he became a Fellow of the College of Physicians and subsequently enjoyed a highly successful and remunerative career as physician to the succeeding sovereigns Edward VI, Mary, and Elizabeth I. The fortune which he acquired he devoted to the benefit of his own college, Gonville Hall. In 1557 he secured for it a new charter, and by endowing it with real estate, raised it in rank from a Hall to a College under the new name of Gonville and Caius College. He provided it with new buildings and endowed it with fellowships and scholarships, of which two were expressly designed to further the study of medicine and, as such, unique in the University. In 1564 he made further provision for medical education within the College, securing from Queen Elizabeth I a special charter to allow it to receive annually for dissection the bodies of two criminals executed in the town or county of Cambridge. Another benefaction came in 1572, when Archbishop Matthew Parker endowed the College with a special scholarship in medicine. This scholarship provided the holder with free lodging and tuition over a period of six years, that is, over the whole of his medical career, and with an annual remuneration of £3 0s. 8d. The holder was required to spend the first three years in the study of 'subjects useful to medicine', and the second three in the study of medicine itself. It was restricted to 'able, learned and worthy youths' born in Kent and educated in Canterbury. At the beginning of the Michaelmas Term, 1593, Harvey was elected to this scholarship and held it for the next six years.

Doubt has sometimes been expressed as to whether Harvey actually began the study of medicine in Cambridge, or whether he chose this subject only after his arrival in the University of Padua. The doubt seems to have arisen from the apparent contradiction in Sir Charles Scarburgh's Harveian Oration of 1662, for he says in one place that it was in Padua that Harvey determined to excel in medicine, and elsewhere that it was at Cambridge that he 'drank philosophy and medicine from the purest and most rich spring of all'.[1] But Scarburgh also relates how he was once called into consultation over a patient together with six other physicians, including Harvey, all of whom had been undergraduates at Caius, and so it would seem that reasonable opportunities for the study of medicine were available in that College. Furthermore, Harvey spent less than three full academic years in Padua and must, therefore, have completed all his undergraduate, preliminary medical studies before his arrival. Moreover, the terms of the Matthew Parker scholarship clearly stated that its holder had to spend the first three years in the study of subjects 'useful to medicine'. Between 1593 and 1597 we may accordingly be certain that this is what Harvey was doing, and in the summer of 1597 he was given leave to supplicate for his degree as a Bachelor of Arts, the necessary preliminary to a degree in medicine.

The undergraduate arts course at Cambridge was at that time still firmly based in the study of the trivium and quadrivium: grammar, rhetoric and logic, arithmetic, geometry, astronomy and music.[2] To qualify for his Bachelor's degree, the student was required to be in residence for sixteen terms, or four years, to attend specified lectures and to perform certain prescribed academic exercises. Little is known about the organisation of the course or the order in which the subjects were studied, or even their total number. It was, however, laid down in the Statutes of Queen Elizabeth I in 1570, that in his first year a student should attend lectures on rhetoric in which the writings of Quintilian and of Hermogenes and the *Orations* of Cicero were read and discussed. The second and third years were devoted to the study of logic and the explanation of Aristotle's dialectical works and Cicero's *Topics*. In the fourth year, philosophy was studied and the lecturer was required to read with the students the *Problems*, *Ethics* or *Politics* of Aristotle, Pliny or Plato.[3] In addition to these subjects, provision was also made in the Statutes for lectures on mathematics, arithmetic, geometry and astronomy, and the works to be studied were those of Pliny, Strabo or Plato on mathematics, of Tunstall or Cardanus on arithmetic, of Euclid on geometry and of Ptolemy on astronomy. All these works, as well as those prescribed for rhetoric, logic and philosophy, the lecturer was bidden to 'explain in the vulgar tongue according to the capacity and intelligence of his hearers'. Finally, the professor of Greek was expected to translate for the undergraduates the writings either of Homer, Isocrates, Demosthenes or Euripides, or of some other ancient author, and to teach the grammatical constructions together with the properties of the language.

From the end of his first year, when just about to begin the course on logic, the undergraduate was required to attend formal disputations two or three times a week, and during his last two years to take an active part in these scholastic exercises.[4] When he had finished his course of lectures and completed the prescribed number of disputations, he could petition the Congregation of Regent Masters to be admitted to the degree of Bachelor of Arts. A complicated series of examinations

6

then followed. First, he was summoned before the Proctors and Regent Masters in the Schools and there asked a number of questions designed to test the extent of his knowledge. If he passed this oral examination, his College granted him a *supplicat* which was sent to the Senate. If the Senate accepted it, the candidate was given the status of 'questionist', which meant that in a formal, ceremonial disputation held in the Schools, he had to answer to a question put to him by an officer of his own College. When this was successfully accomplished, he had to take part as a 'determining bachelor' in the next full-scale Lenten disputations, which were public and the occasion for the display of the best of the candidate's abilities. After that, if adjudged worthy, he received his degree as Bachelor of Arts.

It is reasonable to suppose that Harvey's years at Cambridge were spent in this manner in lectures and disputations. That he was grounded in Greek and Latin literature is probable, and he certainly read rhetoric, logic and philosophy. How much mathematics and astronomy he studied, we cannot guess, but both at Cambridge and at Padua all these subjects formed part of the course in liberal arts which the intending physician had to follow before beginning his studies of medicine proper. In addition to the University lectures and disputations, we know that at Cambridge in Harvey's time a considerable amount of teaching was given in the Colleges, but as Harvey's tutor, George Estey, was a divine and a lecturer in Hebrew, he is likely to have been responsible only for Harvey's general and moral guidance and not for his tuition. At what stage in his career Harvey began the study of medicine proper, is conjectural. The Statutes of 1570 make provision for lectures in medicine to be given to undergraduates and prescribe the books of Hippocrates or Galen for special study. They also say that medical students, before submitting themselves for the degree of Bachelor of Medicine, shall have studied medicine for at least six years, have been assiduous attendants at lectures in that subject, have seen two anatomies and have taken part in three disputations, twice as a respondent and once as a proponent. If Harvey began to study for his Bachelor's degree in medicine in 1597, after finishing his degree in arts, then he may have attended lectures given by the Regius Professor of Physic, William Burton, M.A., Fellow of King's College, on the texts of Hippocrates and Galen, in particular on Galen's *Ars parva*. He may have attended those of the Linacre lecturer, Thomas Cooke, B.A., Fellow of St John's College, also on the texts of classical medical authors. As there was no 'physic garden' in Cambridge at the time, any lectures on botany or simples would most probably have been confined to the reading of works such as those of Dioscorides. As we know that in the 1580's Dr Timothy Bright was lecturing in Cambridge on therapeutics,[5] it is possible that in Harvey's time similar 'unofficial' lectures were also being given although they are unrecorded. In spite of the provisions made for the holding of anatomies both in the University, where the Regius Professor was supposed to lecture at a public dissection every winter, and in Caius College in particular, there is little evidence to show that such dissections actually took place. Thomas Grimston, M.D. and Fellow of Caius, did indeed undertake a public anatomy with 'great credit to him and to the utmost edification of his audience' two years after Harvey had left Cambridge,[6] and he may have demonstrated to Harvey. That Harvey saw at least one anatomy at Cambridge is evident from the reference which he makes in his *Prelectiones* to the spleen cleft into great lobes and the small liver which he had seen in a 'timid' man 'suspenso mortuo scala Cambridg', but whether this refers to a public dissection of an executed malefactor or to an autopsy on a suicide is not possible to decide from the context. This reference to the 'timid' man who was hanged, an allusion to a scholar who was suffocated by burning coals and the statement that 'Wilkinson of Cambridge ate a pig off the spit', all of which occur in the *Prelectiones*, are the sum total of Harvey's allusions to his years in Cambridge. Nowhere does he give any clue as to what he read, saw or did during that time, nor does he record the names of any of his teachers. If he began to work for his Bachelor's degree in medicine in the autumn of 1597, he certainly went down without having completed the curriculum. Moreover, entries in the Exit Book of Caius College show that he was away from Cambridge from 19 September 1598 unto 13 January 1599, during at least part of which time he was ill. In the following July he again left Cambridge, and was again prevented by illness from returning until 27 October. Three days later he once more left the College, with the intention apparently of returning in the following January, but in fact he never returned.[7] By that time it would seem that he was already in Padua.

The mediocre quality of the medical curriculum at Cambridge is to be ascribed to the fact that it was a literary study of the subject. Even in this respect it was one of the most conservative in outlook in the whole of Europe. Because he was aware of the superiority of medical education on the Continent, John Caius stipulated in the rules governing the medical fellowships which he established at his College in 1558, that those who held them might have leave-of-absence to continue their study of medicine abroad. He mentioned Paris, Montpellier, Bologna, and Padua as suitable universities of excellent reputation. Harvey availed himself of this advice, and, leaving Cambridge without taking any further degree, he arrived in Padua in all probability for the beginning of the Michaelmas Term, November 1599. The exact date of his arrival is unknown, for the matriculation registers for this period no longer exist in the University Archives. The first reference to his presence in Padua occurs in August 1600, when he was elected Councillor for the English Nation in the Jurist university.[8] From this certain deductions can be made.

It has in the past caused some surprise that Harvey should thus figure in the Jurist university when he was in fact a student of medicine. The explanation lies in the structure of the University of Padua. Towards the second half of the fourteenth century, the *Universitas studiorum* of Padua was divided into two separate universities, that of the Jurists, the *Universitas iuristarum*, and that of the Artists, that is of the philosophers, theologians and physicians, the *Universitas artistarum*. Each *Universitas* was autonomous with its own organisation and administrative officials. Unlike Oxford and Cambridge, whose governance was vested in the Regent Masters, both universities of Padua were nominally governed by the student body. Each was administered by a Rector and his various assessors and councillors, all of whom were elected annually by the students. Both these student councils had power to treat with the Republic of Venice in all matters of University business. But their power in this respect was, by the beginning of the seventeenth century, more nominal than real. They still had the right to suggest names for appointment to some of the lectureships, and on occasion did so, but such suggestions were always subject to approval and confirmation by the Doge himself. In fact, appointments and matters of University policy were really in the hands of the *Riformatori* (three members of the Venetian Senate who were citizens of Padua), who had been established as a committee by Venice in 1517. Their decisions, made sometimes in consultation with the student body and sometimes with the professors, governed the actual working of the University as a whole. They became responsible for the financial affairs of the University and consequently they, and not the students, paid the salaries

9

of the professors and lecturers. The Rectors of the Jurists and of the Artists were responsible for the details of the administration within their respective universities, and for the maintenance of order and discipline among the students. Within the framework of the two universities, the students were organised according to their Nations, and each Nation elected a representative, a Councillor, to serve with the Rector. With the details of this organisation we are not concerned, but it is important to remember that while all the twenty-two Nations were represented in the Jurist university, only seven were included in the university of the Artists, and neither the English nor the Scottish Nation was among these seven.[9] When, therefore, Harvey was elected Councillor for the English Nation in the Jurist university, it does not mean that he was a member of that university, but simply that he was chosen to represent the English students of the whole *Universitas studiorum*, Artists and Jurists alike, in the only place in which they could be represented. As a medical student, Harvey was, of course, a member of the university of the Artists. His election as Councillor does not prove, as has sometimes been supposed, that he had not by then decided to read medicine; nor does it prove that he was an outstanding student held in great esteem by his countrymen. Though this may be so, a more likely explanation is that in 1600 there were not many Englishmen in Padua who qualified for election.

A Councillor for the English and Scottish Nations first appears in the records of the University of Padua about 1330. Later the two Nations were separated and no Englishman was allowed to supply the office of the Scot. When no suitable Englishman was available, the German Nation had the right to elect one of its members as Councillor for the English. During the first half of the sixteenth century, there were many years in which the English Councillor was not English, but in the second half of the century these occasions became more rare. What happened in the year preceding Harvey's election is not quite clear. A certain 'Rubertus Neurotus' was duly elected on 1 August 1599. On 5 August, Andreas Calafati, doubtfully an Englishman, is named as his substitute. By the following March, the office was vacant and of three substitutes who appear later in the year only one, Alexander Tannus (? Tanner) seems to have been English. Harvey was elected on 1 August 1600 and re-elected on 1 August 1601. He was succeeded in August 1602 by Peter Mounsel, and in 1603 by Robert Willobe (Willoughby). In that year, 1603, the Englishman Simon Fox was permitted, *per gratiam non iure*, to hold office for the Scottish Nation as the two Nations were then united under one King. These three men were all witnesses to Harvey's doctoral diploma.

According to the Statutes of the University of Padua printed in 1600, a student was eligible for election as Councillor only after he had completed two full years in a *studium generale*, and had spent at least one year in the University of Padua. For Harvey to have fulfilled both these conditions by August 1600, which was the end of the academic year, he should have arrived in Padua about the beginning of the Michaelmas Term in November 1599, a supposition which fits reasonably well with the date at which he is known to have left Cambridge. In addition to the residence qualification, a Councillor was further required to be one who, for at least a year before election, had not been a pedagogue or a practising surgeon, who had not lived at the charge of any doctor or citizen of Padua, and who was not a debtor to the University or to any of its officers. None of these qualifications was relevant in Harvey's case. It is to be presumed that he studied at Padua at his father's expense, for his Matthew Parker scholarship ended in 1599.

The duties of the Councillor of the English Nation vis-à-vis the two universities are not clearly explained in the Statutes, but it is to be inferred that he served both Rectors when occasion demanded. Harvey was certainly present as Councillor when doctorates were conferred on English students in the university of the Artists. He was present, for instance, on 19 March 1602 when the degree of doctor of medicine was conferred on Thomas Hearne of Lincoln.[10] He possibly attended similar graduations in law, if any Englishman graduated in the Jurist university during his term of office. That there were not very many English among his contemporaries seems probable. Since no matriculation register for the University as a whole survives from this period, or even for the English Nation, certainty is impossible, but Andrich, in 1892, compiled from other sources in Padua a list of English students known to have been at the University. According to this list, their numbers in the academic years 1596 to 1599 totalled sixteen, nine, three and one respectively. For 1600 to 1602, he gives only one name, that of William Harvey, and in the two following years he lists only two and one. Now these numbers are manifestly incorrect in face of the evidence provided by the names of the witnesses of the doctoral diplomas of Hearne and of Harvey himself. However, in support of the conjecture that the English contingent was not numerous, there is the evidence afforded by the matriculation register of the German Nation of the university of the Artists. Although among all the Ultramontane Nations the German is known to have been the largest, only seventeen students matriculated during the period 20 September to 20 December 1599.[11] It is possible that those who witnessed the diplomas were the only English in Padua at that time.[12]

Harvey's first act on arriving in Padua would have been to present himself to the Councillor for the English Nation whose duty it was, within the next ten days, to report his arrival in writing to the Rector of the university of the Artists and to the *massarius* (the keeper of the University Chest), so that arrangements could be made for his matriculation which had to take place within a month of his coming. When the day was fixed, Harvey would have had to go before the Rector and swear to abide by the Statutes of the University and to obey the Rector and his successors. The Rector on this occasion was Joseph Carrara of Brixen, who later, as Syndic and pro-Rector, witnessed Harvey's doctoral diploma. He would have seen Harvey's name inscribed by the University's notary in the matriculation register of the English Nation and also in the two official registers, the one kept by the *massarius*, the other by the notary. For his official matriculation Harvey would have paid 30 *solidi* to the *massarius* for the benefit of the University, and 4 *solidi* to the notary for writing his name.[13] Once matriculated, Harvey would most probably have gone to live in licensed lodgings in the city. Rules and regulations drawn up by the University sought to ensure that both students and lodging-house keepers maintained a mutual respect. The lodging-house keepers were not allowed to raise the price of lodgings during the course of the academic year, but had to abide by the initial agreements made with the students. They were not allowed to turn the students out unless they repaid them in full. On the other hand, the students were expected to stand by the agreements they had made and when they left they were required to surrender the house key. The earliest surviving register of lodging-houses dates from 1647.[14] In it, each lodging-house keeper listed the names and nationalities of the students living in the house, and signed a declaration to the effect that they had no fire-arms but only their swords. The carrying of fire-arms within the city of Padua was forbidden by law. The wearing of swords by students was only allowed in certain circumstances, and then only with the permission of the Rector. It was expressly forbidden when the students attended Congregation. The only exception was the Rector himself who was permitted to go armed by day and by night. In all public places and in the Schools, the students were expected to wear their gowns. They were not allowed to give their books in pawn, nor could any man deprive them of them in payment for debts. If a student fell sick, unless it were of plague, *quod Deus avertat*, one of the medical professors was required to attend him free of charge. Though there were several epidemics of plague in Padua during the sixteenth century and later, the years which Harvey spent there were free from any outbreak. All the students of Padua enjoyed certain privileges and immunities with regard to the legislature of the city, and the rules governing their conduct were, on the whole, very similar to those obtaining at Oxford and Cambridge at the same period. There seems to be little doubt, however, that the student body at Padua was more international than in either of the English universities. Italians from all the different states of Italy, and Germans, including Flemings, Belgians, Dutch, Swiss and Silesians, preponderated, but in addition there were Poles and Russians, Hungarians, Spaniards and French, as well as a small contingent from the British Isles.

Apart from the records of Harvey's election and re-election as Councillor, no other reference to him is known to exist in the Archives of the University. To have any idea, therefore, of the course of his studies at Padua, we have to make use of the Statutes relating to the medical school in his time, of the lists of the lectures, the *Rotuli*, given during his period of residence, and of the information to be derived from his own doctoral diploma. The simplest method is to begin with the end, with the diploma, and to follow back from there the clues which it provides. The diploma itself is now kept in the library of the Royal College of Physicians in London to which it was given in 1764 by the Reverend Osmund Beauvoir, former Fellow of St John's College, Cambridge and Headmaster of Harvey's old school, King's School, Canterbury. How it came into his possession is unknown. It was published in facsimile in 1908, together with a translation.[15]

Harvey's doctorate, granted to him on 25 April 1602, was not an 'official' doctorate of the University of Padua, but an 'unofficial' one, in the sense that it was not granted with full ecclesiastical authority and in the name of the Sacred College of Philosophers and Physicians,[16] but in that of Sigismund de Capilisti, Count Palatine. Both forms of the doctorate were equally valid, but whereas in the former the

13

recipient had to take an oath to the Roman Catholic Church, in the latter no such obligation was imposed. After the Reformation, the number of Protestant students, particularly German, attending the University of Padua increased and the taking of the oath to the Church was an impediment to many. The Pope was unwilling to allow the granting of doctorates without the oath, and the Republic of Venice replied by the invention of an alternative form. In 1597, it was decided that in such cases the professors, instead of meeting at the Sacred College to examine the candidate, should meet in the house of the Count Palatine,[17] that the examination should take place there and the diploma be issued in the Count's name. This practice obtained until 1616, in which year the Collegio Veneti was founded within the University expressly for Protestants, and this body was then empowered to confer 'official' doctorates. Three kinds of doctorates in medical subjects were given in Padua, one was in medicine alone, the second in medicine and philosophy and the third in surgery. Harvey's doctorate was in medicine and philosophy.

Harvey's diploma explains how, when he had replied to all the questions put to him in 'arts and medicine' by the various professors, and had disputed 'docte, eloquenter, laudabiliter et excellenter', he was given authority to practise and to teach medicine and to enjoy all the privileges enjoyed by the masters and doctors of the Schools of Paris, Cambridge, Oxford, Padua, Bologna, Perugia, Basel, Vienna and Ingolstadt, and was thereupon invested with the insignia of a doctor. Thomas Minadous, professor of the Extra-Ordinary Practice of Medicine handed to him some books of philosophy and medicine, first closed and then open, slipped a golden ring on his finger, set upon his head the doctor's cap in sign of the crown of virtue, and gave him the kiss of peace and the magistral benediction. All this was done in the presence of the two Syndics, Joseph Carrara of Brixen of the university of the Artists, and Peter Buarno of Brixen of the university of the Jurists as pro-Rectors of the respective universities, and a number of English then in Padua: Anthony Fortescue, Richard Willoughby, Matthew Lister, Peter Mounsel, Simon Fox and Robert Darcey.[18] In addition to the Count Palatine, Joseph Carrara and the notary, the diploma was signed by the four professors who had examined Harvey: Hieronymus Fabricius ab Aquapendente, Thomas Minadous, George Raguseus and Julius Casserius.[19]

The assumption that Harvey's examiners were also his teachers does not seem unwarrantable. References to Minadous and Casserius occur in his own writings, and in his *De generatione* he acknowledged his debt to Fabricius as being second only to that to Aristotle: 'in chief, of all the *Ancients*, I follow *Aristotle*; and of later Writers, *Hieronymus Fabricius ab Aquapendente*, Him as my *General*, and this as my *Guide*.' What these various professors were teaching during the years that Harvey was in Padua can to a certain extent be ascertained from various books and documents in the Archives of the University of Padua and elsewhere.

When Harvey arrived in Padua, Fabricius was nearly seventy. He had been appointed by decree of the Doge to succeed Gabriel Falloppius as reader in anatomy and lecturer in surgery on 11 April 1565. The Paduan school of anatomy was already one of the most famous in Europe. It owed its initial renown to Vesalius who had been recognised by his contemporaries from the beginning of his career in Padua as an outstanding young man. Such was his excellence in anatomy that in 1543 it was said of him that 'in our time the subject will be deemed to have been made illustrious by him.'[20] Realdus Columbus, who succeeded him in 1544 ,was also an anatomist of more than ordinary competence, and his discoveries were to be of capital importance for Harvey. Columbus left Padua in 1547, and after an interval of three years during which no appointment was made, he was succeeded, in September 1550, by Gabriel Falloppius. Falloppius combined the lectureship in surgery and anatomy with one in simples, that is botany and materia medica, discussed from a theoretical standpoint. He died on 9 October 1562, 'immatura morte praereptus'; he was not then forty. For two years no appointment was made, but various people undertook the lectures and the dissections. In 1564, the students chose one of these whom they liked and formally requested the Doge to confirm his appointment, but the request was not favourably received for it was thought that he had not come up to expectations. Instead, the *Riformatori* proposed the appointment of Fabricius ab Aquapendente, who had also been teaching and demonstrating during the interim period and had proved himself to be most skilled in dissecting and a capable teacher of anatomy. Periodically his appointment was renewed, each time with an increase in salary until 24 February 1601, when, to mark the fact that he had been teaching in the University for forty years[21] he was given the honorific title of *Professor Supraordinarius* and a pension for life. He did not, however, retire from teaching until November 1613. He died on 31 May 1619, aged about 86.

It was in 1584, after his third re-appointment to the lectureship, that Fabricius's academic status was raised to equal that of an Ordinary Professor of Medicine of the first rank, and the emphasis of his teaching was shifted from surgery to anatomy, so that he became in effect professor of anatomy. (It was not until 1609 that, by a decree of the Doge, the chair of anatomy was divorced from surgery.) In 1584 also, he was admitted to membership of the Sacred College of Philosophy and Medicine, in spite of the protests of some of his colleagues, who were unwilling that a mere professor of anatomy and a surgeon should share their privileges. His election meant that from then on he had equal rights with the professors of the Theory and Practice of Medicine to examine candidates for medical degrees. In that year also an anatomy theatre was constructed for the first time indoors. Until then it had been the custom to build each year a temporary wooden structure which was removed at the end of the course. This was expensive – the bedellus reported in July 1583, that he had spent 21 ducats, 3 livres and 12 sous on the anatomy theatre in that year – and, being out-of-doors, it had all the obvious disadvantages. The structure erected in 1584 on the advice of Laurentius Massa, the secretary of the *Riformatori*, was still wooden and dismountable, but it was housed in one of the upper rooms of the University building, known as *Il Bò*, to which the medical faculty had moved in 1542. In 1594, the famous anatomy theatre of Fabricius, as it is now called, was constructed in an upper room in the same University building where it may be seen to this day.[22] It was there that Harvey as a student attended the anatomical demonstrations of Fabricius.

According to the rules for the holding of anatomies laid down in the Statutes of the University published in Venice in 1589, the task of the lecturer in surgery on these occasions was limited to making the incisions and dissecting the body, while one professor of medicine read the text of the *Anatomia* of Mondino di Luzzi and another repeated it sentence by sentence, showed what was described and verified the statements with reference to the cadaver. By this date, however, there is little doubt that this practice had been abandoned. Vesalius certainly both dissected and commented on his findings, and although he may not have been the initiator of this reform, from his time onwards the ancient custom disappeared. In fact, in the spring of 1553, Falloppius tried to re-introduce it, but the students created such an uproar that the Schools had to be shut, and afterwards Falloppius undertook all the anatomies alone. It was in Falloppius's time also that anatomy is said to have 'flourished greatly'. So popular did the subject become that not only were the statutory public dissections held regularly, but also private dissections were frequently undertaken: 'non publicae modo, sed privatae quoque exercitationes passim habebantur.' The enthusiasm of the students was so great that, when subjects for dissection were lacking, they took to robbing graves until the Venetian Senate passed a decree imposing severe penalties for such conduct.[23] A year or so later, in 1555, as the supply of bodies still did not meet the demand, the anatomical school was given permission to receive them not only from the domain of the city of Padua, but from the whole territory of the Venetian Republic.

Fabricius himself performed both public and private anatomies. He was a highly skilled dissector and anatomist, an excellent teacher and popular with the students. In an official letter from the Doge, written in 1589, it is said that during the twenty-four years in which he had been teaching he had spared himself none of the fatigues attendant upon his charge, but had taught with great profit and advantage to the students who crowded to his lectures and demonstrations. Much is known about his teaching, not from official University sources but from the Acts of the German Nation, a record of events which was kept by the German Councillor.[24] The purpose of his course was a general survey of the anatomy of the whole human body, and it was frequently supplemented by a detailed study of special organs and by dissections of animals of different kinds. In order to give the students a better understanding of what they saw at the formal anatomies, it was proposed in 1583, that a new series of lectures on anatomical method should be instituted. Fabricius is known to have given this course at least four times during his career. The fourth occasion was during the academic year 1600–01, when Harvey was a student in Padua and could have been present. If he arrived during the Michaelmas Term 1599, then he was there when the students of the German Nation obtained from Fabricius a promise to perform for them during that winter both a general anatomy and a special dissection of the lower belly and to give them some specialised teaching in surgery and a demonstration of all the surgical instruments employed. This promise Fabricius abundantly fulfilled. In January 1600, a period of particularly cold weather, he gave a 'most praiseworthy' course. He began with human and comparative osteology, paying particular attention to the bones of birds. This he followed with a long and detailed anatomy lasting a number of days and using for the purpose three bodies, two male and one female. Finally, he gave a separate dissection of the eye. In the same year, in the autumn, in addition to the lectures in the Schools on anatomical method already referred to, he demonstrated in the Anatomy Theatre the anatomy of the foetus of a horse and of a sheep, no human subjects being available for dissection. In January 1601, when a body had been procured, he gave a complete human anatomy which is said to have tired him considerably, but recovering, he proceeded to the demonstration of many surgical operations. A letter from the Rector to the *Riformatori*, dated 29 July 1601, says that in this academic year Fabricius had given his lectures every day, both working days and holy days, without interruption from the commencement until Easter. But in the following November, he was again putting off the requests of the students for anatomies, as he had many times in the past, with fair words and golden promises, and he does not seem to have performed another public anatomy until after Harvey had taken his doctor's degree.

The *Rotuli*, or lists containing the names of the professors and the subjects on which they were lecturing and the times of the lectures, though extant for many of the years from the sixteenth century onwards, are wanting for two of the three years that Harvey was in Padua. The one which does exist for 1601–02 unfortunately only gives the names of the professors and their salaries, the hours at which they were lecturing but not the subjects of their lectures. From other lists, however, we know that Fabricius was in the habit of lecturing each year on one of the following subjects: Of similar and dissimilar parts and their actions; Of fractures and luxations; Of tumours; Of particular diseases. His lectures, as opposed to his demonstrations, are not often mentioned in the Acts of the German Nation and opinion as to their value seems to have been divided. In January 1581, Fabricius promised to lecture on tumours, fractures and luxations. 'How he acquitted himself on that occasion on the treatment of tumours,' wrote the German Councillor, 'you know well; he never got as far as the teaching on fractures, and as for luxations, he omitted those entirely.' Yet it was his lectures on surgery which were pirated and printed in Frankfurt from a student's notes in 1592. There, in the introduction, we read that he taught surgery 'incredibili multorum admiratione'. This book is said to correspond well enough with a manuscript in the library of the University of Cracow which contains the notes written by four Polish students who attended Fabricius's

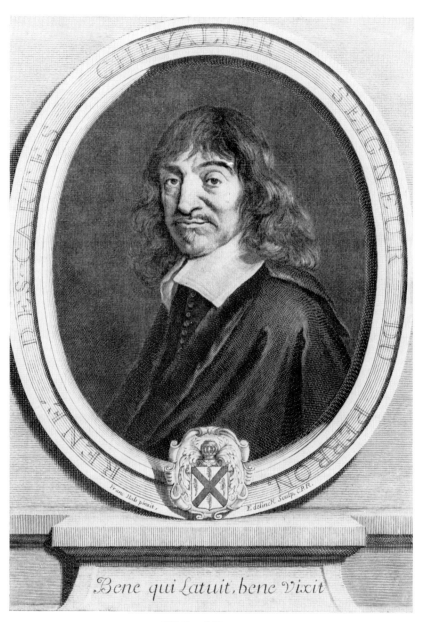

III René Descartes

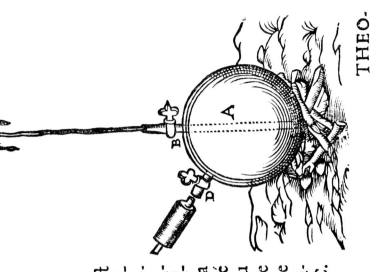

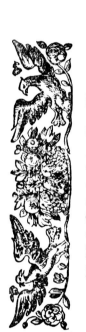

THEORESME V.

L'eau montera par aide du feu, plus haut que son niveau.

E troisiesme moyen de faire monter, est par l'aide du feu, dont il se peut faire diuerses machines, i'en donneray icy la demonstration d'vne. Soit vne balle de cuiure marquée A. bien soudée tout à l'entour, à laquelle il y aura vn soufpiral marqué D. par ou lon mettra l'eau, & aussi vn tuyau marqué B. C. qui sera soudé en haut de la balle, & le bout C. approchera pres du fond, sans y toucher, apres faut emplir ladite balle d'eau par le soufpiral, puis le bien reboucher & le mettre sur le feu, alors la chaleur donnant contre la-dire balle, fera monter toute l'eau, par le tuyau B. C.

IV *The expulsion of water from a heated sphere: a process similar to Descartes's explanation of the expulsion of blood by the heart*

lectures on surgery in 1580-1. That is the very year in which the German Councillor had passed so acid a comment. In December 1606, however, the Councillor had nothing but the highest praise for Fabricius's surgical lectures and demonstrations.

More important for Harvey's future work than the lectures on surgery were Fabricius's anatomical demonstrations and physiological discussions. In addition to the formal instruction which they gave in the University, most of the professors and lecturers at this time taught privately. Fabricius was no exception, and that Harvey worked privately with him might perhaps be inferred from a passage in *De generatione* where he says that once, in the spring, he had made certain observations on two hens and a cock 'to prepare a defence for Fabricius', *ut hic Fabricio patrocinium parem.*[25] (Perhaps he was defending Fabricius's theories on fecundation from adverse criticisms.) There are indeed a number of similarities between Harvey and Fabricius, both in their manner of work and in their approach to the subject of their study. One characteristic which they seem to have had in common was the capacity for minute and careful observation, and the patience which this entails. Precise attention to detail marks both their works. An interest in comparative anatomy was shared by both of them. Whereas Vesalius had focused his attention on human anatomy and dissected monkeys, dogs and pigs only as substitutes for the human body and not for their own sake, Fabricius saw the value of a comparative study, and dissected a very great variety of creatures. Nor was Fabricius interested in anatomy only for the sake of anatomy, but for the light which this study could throw on the problems of action and function. In the foreword to *De voce*, published in Venice in 1600, Fabricius criticised Vesalius for neglecting certain aspects of his subject, for confining himself almost entirely to minute description of the parts and saying practically nothing of their action and function. It is quite obvious from Harvey's *Prelectiones* that mere anatomical description was not his chief interest. He is far more concerned with the action and function of the parts. In modern terminology, he is not primarily an anatomist, but a physiologist.

All the anatomical dissections which Fabricius performed and all the discussions which arose from them, were directed to the fulfilment of his life-long ambition, the publication of a work to be called *Totius animalis fabricae theatrum*, illustrated with coloured plates in natural size, each accompanied by a black-and-white engraving. He began to prepare these plates at least by 1591 and some three hundred were eventually made. The greater part of these still exist in the Bibliotheca Marciana in Venice, for he bequeathed them at his death to the Republic with a request that they might be preserved in the State Library. The aim of this vast project was to supplement the work of Vesalius. He criticised Vesalius not only for his failure to describe the action and the function of the parts, but for being obscure and long-winded in style, too prolix and not infrequently irrelevant, and moreover, incomplete, because many discoveries had been made since his time by anatomists such as Realdus Columbus, Falloppius, Eustachius, Jasolinus, and even by Fabricius himself. Over the years he worked on various parts of this programme and wrote diverse treatises on specialised subjects. These he allowed to accumulate, subjecting each one to long and careful criticism in the hope that thereby error would be avoided.

> If it surprises anyone that I am issuing only one part at a time, and not producing the whole work at once, let him know that this plan ensures far greater accuracy in the individual pamphlets, since time is taken for revision, and the facts are carefully considered. This may cause delay but it affects very markedly the finish of the whole work, which becomes in consequence both intrinsically finer and also more useful to the reader.

In the event only a few of these treatises were written and published, and Fabricius died without having fulfilled his ambition. His preoccupation with these 'monographs' is reflected in the subjects he chose for his special demonstrations. A constantly recurring theme was animal generation in all its different aspects. Anatomies of foctuses, human and animal, are frequently mentioned as special demonstrations. He dissected living gravid animals of various kinds. He showed the uterus and placenta of a pregnant woman; he demonstrated the genital organs of both sexes. All these are dissections specially mentioned in the Acts of the German Nation. His interest in this subject was certainly shared by Harvey who may indeed have learnt it from him. But as we are not concerned with Harvey's work on the generation of animals, his debt to Fabricius on this score can be passed over.[26] What is important for the present purpose is to ascertain, if possible, what Fabricius taught concerning the movement of the heart and blood.

It was in 1603, after Harvey had left Padua, that Fabricius published his treatise on the valves of the veins, *De venarum ostiolis*. Here he claimed to have seen them for the first time in 1574:

As we are about to discuss these valves, we must first express our surprise at the way in which they have escaped the notice of Anatomists, both of our own and earlier generations: so much so that not only have they never been mentioned, but no one even set eye on them till 1574, when to my great delight I saw them in the course of my dissection.[27]

Salomon Alberti in his *Tres orationes*, printed in Nuremberg in 1585, gave an account of the valves with full acknowledgement to Fabricius, but he also mentioned that they had been pointed out to Vesalius by Giambattista Canano in 1544. With these and other rival claims to priority we are not concerned; what is important is to know if Fabricius was in the habit of demonstrating these valves to the students in Padua. Alberti says, on hearsay evidence (*fertur*), that Fabricius showed them publicly for the first time at the beginning of 1579, and that during the course of the same year, he too had shown them to his students in their anatomy theatre at Wittemberg, where he had been professor since 1573. Confirmation of Alberti's statement comes from Caspar Bauhin of Basel who had been a student in Padua for approximately eighteen months from October 1577. During this period he saw seven complete anatomies, some of which were public dissections performed by Fabricius and others private in which he himself had assisted.[28] It was in the course of one of these anatomies by Fabricius in the winter of 1578-9 that he saw the valves in the veins. In 1590 Bauhin published from Basel his anatomical textbook, *De corporis humani fabrica, Libri IIII*, in which, having said that Fabricius had demonstrated the valves for 'more than sixteen years', he describes them in terms which may well derive directly from the teaching of Fabricius.[29] That Fabricius continued to demonstrate the valves in subsequent years is more than likely, and consequently that Harvey saw such a demonstration is almost certain. If Harvey saw the demonstration, then he also heard the interpretation of their use, and this is explained by Fabricius in accordance with the Galenic notion of the movement of the blood:

My theory is that Nature has formed them to delay the blood to some extent, and to prevent the whole mass of it from flooding into the feet, or hands and fingers, and collecting there. Two evils are thus avoided, namely, under-nutrition of the upper parts of the limbs, and a permanently swollen condition of the hands and feet. Valves were made, therefore, to ensure a really fair distribution of the blood for the nutrition of the various parts. . . . The activity which Nature has here devised is strangely like that which artificial means have produced in the

21

machinery of mills. Here engineers put certain hindrances in the water's way so that a large quantity of it may be kept back and accumulate for the use of the milling machinery.... In like manner Nature labours in the veins by means of valves, here singly, there in pairs, the veins themselves representing the channels for the streams.... valves are placed in veins less with a view to causing a pooling and storing of blood before the oblique mouths of the branches than with a view to checking it on its course and preventing the whole mass of it from slipping headlong down and escaping.

Bauhin, in 1590, had given a similar explanation: that the use of the valves in the veins of the arms and legs was to prevent the blood from falling impetuously into the lower parts of the limbs, and so overwhelming them with too much nourishment while the upper parts were starved. By delaying the blood, the valves allowed a further concoction to take place in the blood so that it was more perfectly fitted for its work of nutrition. This explanation is not entirely in accordance with Galen's teaching but does not contradict it. Galen had got round the difficulty of the idea of the blood falling down into the lower parts of the limbs, by attributing an 'attractive' power to the parts, so that the blood went where and when it was required.

While wondering why other anatomists had not noticed the valves, Fabricius explains how he had seen them during a demonstration of the veins:

> For in the bare veins exposed to view, but still uninjured, the valves in a manner display themselves. Nay more, when assistants pass a ligature round the limbs preparatory to blood-letting, valves are quite obviously noticeable in the arms and legs of the living subject. And, indeed, at intervals along the course of the veins certain knotty swellings are visible from the outside; these are caused by the valves. In some people, in fact, such as porters and peasants, they appear to swell up like varices....

Support for his belief that the valves slowed the impetus of the blood was found by Fabricius in the following experiment:

> That the blood is slowed by the valves, evident even without this from their actual construction, can be tested by anyone either in the exposed veins of the cadaver, or in the living subject if he passes a ligature round the limbs as in blood-letting. For if one tries to exert pressure on the blood, or to push it along by rubbing from above downwards, one will clearly see it held up and delayed by the valves. This indeed was the way in which I was led to an observation of such nature.

In 1628 Harvey was to use a very similar experiment to a vastly different purpose. It is strange that Fabricius did not notice that, when the pressure was released, the blood flowed *upwards* to refill the vein. It may well be that it was the observation of this phenomenon that first puzzled Harvey. But Fabricius was so firmly persuaded of the truth of the Galenic doctrine that he saw what he expected to see. If he did notice the blood returning, he could have explained it as an observation made at the moment of the reflux of the blood, and for this he was prepared. Though his descriptions of the valves are for the most part precise and accurate, he failed to realise their competence, a further fact of whose importance Harvey subsequently became aware. There is no indication from the text of his treatise that Fabricius tried the effect of pushing against the valves with a probe. Though Bauhin in 1590 refers to the use of a probe, it is merely to remark that if you blow into a vein at the same time inserting a probe, you will see the valves distend like bladders.[30] Fabricius believed that the valves were deliberately arranged not to occlude the lumen of the veins:

> Nature has so placed the valves that in every case the higher valves are on the opposite side of the vein to those immediately below them. . . . In this way the lower valves always delay whatever slips past the upper ones, but meanwhile the passage of the blood is not blocked.

Galen's theory concerning the movement of the arterial blood and the structure of the arteries seemed to Fabricius to support his explanation of the valves in the veins:

> Arteries, on the other hand, had no need of valves, either to prevent distension – the thickness of their coat suffices – or to delay the blood – an ebb and flow goes on continually within them.

Further evidence that Fabricius was to a considerable extent an orthodox Galenist is not lacking. In *De formato foetu*, he adopts the Galenic account of the foetal blood. This work was published in 1604, but was already in process of being written in 1592 and is almost certainly based on his lectures and demonstrations. His description of the umbilical vessels, the ductus venosus, the foramen ovale and the ductus arteriosus is essentially accurate, and on certain points Fabricius corrects Galen saying that 'his opinion does not agree with dissection'. But in the interpretation of these anatomical facts, Fabricius adopts Galen's idea that the foetus lives the life of a plant and needs for its growth only blood, which provides its food, and vital spirit which assists in the concoction of this food. The blood, derived from the maternal liver, is carried into the foetus through the umbilical vein, and the vital spirit, derived from the maternal heart, enters through the umbilical artery. The liver and the heart of the foetus have no part of their own to play in the development of the foetus, or, as Galen puts it, have no public office to perform.

> Since the foetal heart beats of its own nature and the character of its temperament, it beats to preserve its own individual existence, and all the arteries connected with the great artery likewise pulsate in accordance with the heart beat. This, however, is not a public office of the heart, because this pulsation of the heart and arteries is useful in attracting some vital blood from the uterine arteries into the heart and the arteries of the whole body by way of the umbilical arteries. . . . blood is not supplied by the foetal heart to all its arteries, but the mother supplies it to both the heart and arteries of the foetus.

This contention, Fabricius says, is proved by Galen's experiment of ligating the umbilical vessels at the navel, whereupon the foetal arteries cease to pulsate.

> Now, if in the foetus the vital blood proceeded from the heart into the whole body as it does in the adult, certainly neither the arteries of the whole body nor the heart would suffer any harm when the veins and arteries at the umbilicus were ligated.

At the end of chapter 2, Fabricius sums up his doctrine on the subject and gives an account, which is Galenic, of the way in which the nutriment, or chyle, is distributed throughout the body of the foetus:

> Now while the foetus is being carried in the uterus it is governed as follows. Aliment in the form of blood is sucked up from the uterus, as if from the ground, by the chorionic vessels acting as roots; next, it is carried to the liver, as to a trunk, so that it may be distributed from that point to the whole foetus, which corresponds to the entire plant, by the extensions of the vena cava and portal vein, which serve as the branches. Similarly, when the foetus has been born and its governance and its veins have been altered, aliment, chyle in this case, is sucked up from the stomach and intestines as if from the ground by the roots of the portal vein, which are the mesenteric veins acting like the roots of a plant. The chyle first reaches the trunk of the portal vein and is then transmitted to its branches distributed throughout the liver. By them it is carried

into the substance of the liver, so that there the chyle may be changed into blood, the true and appropriate nutriment of animals. Thereafter, the blood is taken up by the roots of the vena cava which spread throughout the liver, and is carried to its convex portion, as if to a trunk, whence it is distributed by all the branches of the vena cava through the entire body for its nutrition and the restoration of lost substance.

In chapter 8, Fabricius comes to the Uses of the Vessels of the Heart. Here he follows Galen and explains that the vessel on the right side of the foetal heart is the foramen of the vena cava leading into the right 'ventricle' (*sc.* atrium), and that it opens into the pulmonary vein. The vessel on the left is a short, arterial branch emerging from the aorta as it leaves the heart, and communicating with the pulmonary artery which leads to the lungs. Both vessels are closed after birth; the right is closed by the valve at its base which is glued shut, and the left wastes away and is thus closed. As the lungs do not perform the office of respiration in the foetus, they receive the blood for their nourishment through the pulmonary vein and vital spirit through the pulmonary artery.

At this date there was considerable controversy on the question of the origin of the veins. Aristotle had taught that they arose from the heart, Galen and most of the medical anatomists that they came from the liver, Vesalius that the liver was formed from them. Fabricius supported Galen. On at least four different occasions, in 1576, 1578-9, 1586 and 1593, the German Councillor reported that Fabricius had made a special demonstration of the liver showing how the veins arose from it. According to a letter written by Christopher Schilling and relating to the winter of 1578-9, Fabricius, after a very detailed anatomy of the lower belly during which he paid particular attention to the distribution in the liver of the portal vein and the vena cava, showed the students that the liver was the 'principium non tantum dispensationis, sed etiam generationis venarum' (not only the source from which the veins were distributed throughout the body, but from which they took their origin). In addition to the vena cava and the portal vein, Fabricius showed how the umbilical vein grew out from the liver, as plants do from the earth, and he maintained that in the foetus this vein served the office of the portal vein ('l'ufficio della porta'). From this it is clear that between 1578 and 1604 Fabricius had not changed his opinion concerning the blood supply to the foetus. Though he is not known to have given a detailed anatomy of the liver while Harvey was in Padua, a discussion of it must have come into the general anatomies. The truth of this Galenic doctrine on the origin of the veins was to be called in question by Harvey in his *Prelectiones* of 1616 before the death of Fabricius. 'Nor is the liver the beginning of the veins, for the veins exist in the embryo and in the egg before the liver.'[31]

In addition to his belief that the arterial blood ebbed and flowed incessantly in the arteries, Fabricius held that the arteries arose from the heart, and he subscribed to the Galenic belief in the association between respiration and the action of the heart. This association he summarised in *De formato foetu*, chapter 8, where he writes of the lungs in the adult:

> First they take up and receive through the trachea the air drawn in by breathing. This is then carried by the heart-beat through the venous artery [*sc.* pulmonary vein] into the left chamber of the heart to be concocted and changed into vital spirit, and to furnish refrigeration to the heart. Through the third vessel, however, which is called the arterial vein [*sc.* pulmonary artery], the lungs are nourished by the purest and thinnest blood.

In his treatise *De respiratione et eius instrumentis*, printed in 1615, Fabricius explains how, since air is necessary for life and the heart is the fountain and origin of life, air must be necessary for the heart. The heart has three actions of its own: pulsation, passion,[32] and, because it is the fountain of heat or vital spirit, the distribution of this heat or vital spirit throughout the body. Air is necessary to maintain the heat of the heart at the right temperature, neither too hot nor too cold, to refrigerate its innate fire. The pulsation of the heart consists in its dilatation and contraction. While the heart is dilating, it draws in the air which cools the innate heat; while it is contracting, it drives out fuliginous vapours. From all this it is clear enough that Fabricius believed and taught the Galenic theory of the heart's action and of the movement of the blood.

Some six years before Fabricius was appointed to the lectureship in Padua, there was printed in Venice at the end of 1559, the posthumous work of Realdus Columbus, *De re anatomica*, in which the pulmonary transit of the blood was described. Fabricius certainly knew of this book, for in his treatise *De respiratione*, he refers to Columbus's opinion on the use of the diaphragm in order to contradict it and to say 'in this Realdus was deceived.'[33] But he makes no mention in any of his books of Columbus's work on the nature of systole and diastole of the heart or on the pulmonary transit of the blood. Whether he referred to it in his anatomies is debatable. As he was a firm believer in the Galenic

26

doctrine of the existence of pores in the interventricular septum of the heart, Fabricius had no need to explain the presence of blood in the left ventricle by supposing that it arrived by way of the lungs. On occasion, however, his teaching on the intraventricular pores does seem to have aroused a certain scepticism among the students. In a letter written on 26 January 1576, the German Councillor, Peter Monaw, said that at the end of the general course in anatomy, which had then just finished, Fabricius showed the students the origin of the veins in the liver and 'by means of a probe, the passage between the two cardiac ventricles, whose existence (already denied by Vesalius) many doubt, and this gave rise to a lively and interesting discussion'.

However great Harvey's debt to Fabricius may have been in general terms, he did not get from him at Padua the slightest hint as to the correct interpretation of the valves of the veins. He did not learn from him the truth concerning systole and diastole of the heart nor the fact of the pulmonary transit of the blood. It is true that their interests were similar. Both wrote on the generation of animals. Fabricius wrote a treatise on respiration; Harvey intended to write one. In fact, Fabricius's work on the muscles concerned in respiration was repeated by Harvey, as is clear from his *Prelectiones*. It is interesting to notice that in the discussion as to whether or not the sternum and the cartilages have any specific part to play in the movements of respiration, Fabricius says that this is not clear in man, because the very slight movements of the cartilages depend upon those of the diaphragm, and consequently it is usual to say that the sternum and cartilages are not of great importance for respiration,

> as we proved in 1599, when we found a cadaver in which the cartilages were wanting and the ribs osseous to the very sternum, which itself was without any division; and this, which is commonly known as *petto integro*, is, I think, a sure sign that in man the movement of the sternum and of the cartilages of the ribs is not very necessary.

It is just possible that Harvey saw this demonstration. But Fabricius was interested in more than the movement of the muscles concerned in respiration; he was fascinated by the mechanics of all muscular movement. In 1614 he published one treatise on muscles and another on joints, in which he dealt with the structure, action and utilities of muscle and joint respectively. In 1618 he published his treatise *De motu locali animalium secundum totum* in which he discussed all manner of animal progression, that is to say, walking in general, walking of bipeds, of quadrupeds and multipeds, flying, swimming and crawling. Harvey too was interested in this problem of muscular movement as is evident from the notes which he was writing in 1627 for a treatise he never published entitled *De motu locali animalium*. In spite of its title, it has little to do with Fabricius's treatise of the same name, but it does owe a large debt to his earlier three-part treatise on muscle. Neither Fabricius nor Harvey made any lasting contribution to this particular field of study, though Harvey was right in his deduction that the essential contractile element in muscle is fleshy fibre. The development of the lens and the microscope was not, in 1627, sufficiently advanced to provide Harvey with the tools necessary to push his studies further. The subject had to wait for another forty years, and it is to Nicholas Steno and his *Elementorum myologiae specimen*, published in 1667, that credit must be given for the first beginnings of the analysis of muscular contraction.

The last of the examiners to sign Harvey's doctoral diploma, being inferior in academic rank to the others, was Julius Casserius of Piacenza. As a boy, it is said, he had been a servant to Fabricius, but later he became his pupil and assistant, and taught both surgery and anatomy in the University of Padua. Much of his teaching, however, seems to have been unofficial. He is first mentioned in the Acts of the German Nation in 1586, when he gave a private anatomy for the German students at his own house. It lasted from 11 to 23 February and afterwards Casserius demonstrated the chief surgical operations, As he held no official appointment and was not in receipt of a salary from the University, but was paid by the students in money or kind, it is difficult to know the extent of Casserius's teaching, but that it went on every year seems a reasonable supposition.[34] He himself says that he gave an anatomy in 1593 before an audience largely composed of German students. By that time his plans for publishing his anatomical writings were well advanced and this anatomy was attended by the painter, Joseph Mauer, in order to make the drawings to illustrate the books. That Harvey attended his anatomical demonstrations is to be inferred from a reference to him in the *Prelectiones*. There Harvey says that Julius of Piacenza opened a man from whom he removed a great quantity of sanies from an empyema.[35] As far as I know, there is no reference to this in any of Casserius's printed works. Harvey may well either have seen it done, or heard of it direct from Casserius. On 9 May 1601,

28

Casserius was admitted Doctor of Medicine and Philosophy by the Sacred College in Padua, and this may have given him the authority to examine. In the same year, his first anatomical textbook, *De vocis auditusque organis,* was published at Ferrara. It was not, however, until after Harvey left Padua that Casserius was formally entrusted with any of the teaching of Fabricius. Though he had been asked in February 1604 to undertake the public anatomy when Fabricius was ill, the Acts of the German Nation state that in 1605 he had the University's licence to perform private anatomies only. At the beginning of 1609, Fabricius relinquished to him the lectureship in surgery, but continued to hold the chair of anatomy until November 1613. Casserius was then appointed in his place, but in that year refused to hold the formal anatomy in the Anatomical Theatre, preferring to demonstrate in a room in the Collegio Brixiano. He did not consent to perform in the public theatre until January 1614. He died in 1616, three years before Fabricius.

As a surgeon, Casserius is credited with being one of the first to perform the operation of laryngotomy, or tracheotomy; as an anatomist his greatest contribution was made to the field of comparative anatomy. At the anatomies which he gave, he followed the example of Fabricius and divided his time between demonstrating cadavers, dissecting many different kinds of animals and performing vivisections. For example, in the course of the great anatomy lasting five weeks which he gave to the German students in the spring of 1598, he used a monkey, several live dogs and nine cadavers.[36] In January 1614, after dissecting several cadavers, he showed the recurrent nerves in a live dog. In his writings he tries to explain the fabric of man by reference to the lower animals. His investigations in comparative anatomy were the most extensive and the best to have been carried out up to his time, and such they remained for long after his death. He may well have fostered Harvey's interest in the comparative study of anatomy.

Harvey's debt to Padua in the field of anatomy and physiology is abundantly obvious. His training in medicine is more difficult to assess, probably because we know less about him as a physician. It was laid down in the Statutes of the University of Padua, that those wishing to submit themselves for a degree in medicine must have studied that subject for at least three years, attended all the 'ordinary' lectures, disputed publicly with one of the doctors, replied to questions put to them in the Medical Faculty and read lectures publicly in the Schools. In addition, the candidate was expected to have practised medicine for at least one year with a well-known physician and to have visited the sick, 'and if there is any doubt about this, let it stand on his oath, unless he have a formal dispensation'. It is well known that the practice of teaching at the bedside had been introduced into Padua by Giovanni Baptista da Monte, who, in April 1543, taught medical students in the hospital of St Francis. With various interruptions, this practice continued over the years. After one such interruption, in the spring of 1596, the students wrote to the *Riformatori* requesting its resumption. They received a reply to the effect that the professors not only had permission, but indeed an obligation, to give practical instruction to the students as often as they wanted it, provided that it did not coincide with the hours of the formal lectures. From the references which Harvey makes in his *Prelectiones* to cases which he had seen in the hospitals in Italy, it may be presumed that he, like others, was taught clinical medicine in the hospital of St Francis, but we do not know which physician was his teacher.

The extent of Harvey's knowledge of pathology and morbid anatomy, as revealed in all his published works, has, on occasion, aroused a certain amount of comment and speculation as to how he acquired this knowledge. It seems certain that the foundations were laid in Padua. In Cambridge, in Oxford, and in the colleges of Physicians and Barber-Surgeons in London, the subjects for the public anatomies were the bodies of criminals hanged on the gallows. The discovery in them of diseased organs was entirely fortuitous. The University of Padua also, as has been said, made use of similar subjects, but in Padua the total number of bodies dissected seems to have been far greater than anywhere in England, so that one may well ask how these cadavers were obtained and whether they were all criminals who had been hanged. Information on this subject is difficult to obtain. The University records do not mention even every formal anatomy that was held. Other sources, though giving information on some private anatomies, are equally incomplete. Judicial records do not help either. And here another difficulty arises, for although in England hanging was the common form of execution and decapitation reserved for the privileged, in the Republic of Venice beheading was the frequent punishment for infanticide and other kinds of murder, and this reduced the number of subjects suitable for anatomical demonstrations. In an unpublished chronicle by Niccolò de' Rossi, *Listoria di Padova*, which covers the years 1562 to 1621,[37] there is a considerable amount of information on public executions in Padua, but only on one occasion does the writer say that the body was given to the students for an anatomy. That was in March 1599. The body of a young man hanged for murder was taken from the high gallows in the Piazza della Signoria and dragged away tied to a horse's tail and given to the students for an anatomy ('e menato a coda di cavallo il corpo suo fu dato per anatomia alli Scolari'). No other source mentions an anatomy at this date. If the bodies for the formal, public anatomies were those of executed criminals, as is indeed certain, the problem still remains as to where the subjects for the private anatomies were obtained. Despite orders to the contrary, graves were robbed from time to time. It was a practice in which even Vesalius had indulged. To counter rumours that the students stole bodies and after dissecting them threw the remains into the river or gave them to the dogs to eat, it was officially decreed in 1597 that the ancient custom of providing a public funeral for the dissected body should be reinstated. There was, however, one legitimate source of bodies in Padua and that was the hospital of St Francis. The question that is difficult to answer is to what extent it was used. We know that autopsies were carried out on patients who died in that hospital because the German Councillor records that in 1578, Marco de Oddis, first professor of the Extra-Ordinary Theory of Medicine, dissected the bodies of two women who had died there to show the students the diseased organs. If this practice continued, and it is to be believed that it did, it was from autopsies of this kind that the students learned their pathology and morbid anatomy. We have no means of knowing whether bodies used at private anatomies came from this source.

While on this subject of post-mortem examinations, it is interesting to remember that Alessandro Benedetti (1460–1525), who had been professor of anatomy in Padua, pointed out in his book, *Historia corporis humani sive anatomice*, that the practice then obtaining of allowing the medical school to use only the bodies of executed malefactors for the teaching of anatomy, was inadequate for this purpose. He asserted the absolute necessity of finding supplementary material for dissection from other sources. He may have said this for the simple reason that he knew that no student could learn the subject properly by merely attending one or two formal anatomies during the course of his studies. On the other hand, Benedetti had been a pupil of Antonio Benevieni, the Florentine anatomist, who is now considered to be the founder of pathology and morbid anatomy because he published, in 1507, in his

De abditis nonnullis mirandis morborum ac sanitationum causis, accounts of the many post-mortem examinations which he had conducted. Of the value of these autopsies to the medical students, Benedetti may have been fully aware, and perhaps he was partly instrumental in introducing the practice into Padua. This whole question of post-mortem examinations, as opposed to anatomies, has not as yet been investigated and would repay a closer study. At whatever date such examinations became more than rare occurrences, it is certain that by the last quarter of the sixteenth century they were frequently performed, and they were by no means limited to those held in the hospital of St Francis.

The Public Health Department (l'Ufficio della Sanità) had been founded in Venice in 1348 and was established in Padua in 1531, after the death of Benedetti. Besides dealing with regulations regarding food and provisions, street cleaning, apothecaries and their drugs, charlatans and beggars, it supervised cattle and cattle epidemics and was perpetually on guard against the outbreak of plague in the territory of Padua. Because of the ever-present fear of a fresh occurrence of this disease, it forbade the burial of any person dying from unknown causes without a doctor's certificate to prove that the body had been examined and that the cause of death was not plague. The Department maintained a number of physicians at whose orders these examinations were conducted. From 1598 onwards, there exist a number of certificates from physicians testifying to the fact that the patient had died from the expected cause, and that this was not plague. One such certificate given by Thomas Minadous, 'primo prattico dello Studio', existing from the year 1613, testifies that the man in question had died from an acute fever as had been foreseen, and that his death was 'senza sospetto alcuno di male contagiosa imaginabile'. Not all these examinations of the dead were detailed autopsies, and it is not known whether the students attended. But in Padua at this date there was much information available from many different sources on all manner of post-mortem findings, and the examination of the dead was of common occurrence.

Thomas Minadous of Rovigo, who invested Harvey with the insignia of a doctor, had himself been a student at Padua and had taken his doctor's degree in 1576. After a period in the Venetian consulate in the Levant, where he collected material for his history of the Turkish-Persian war, he returned to Italy, and in July 1596 was appointed to the first chair of the Extra-Ordinary Practice of Medicine. During the years in which Harvey was in Padua, Minadous and his colleagues, Alexander

Vigontiae and John Peter Peregrinus, were engaged in lecturing on Particular diseases from the head to the heart, Particular diseases from the heart downwards, and Fevers. The professors of the Ordinary Practice of Medicine, Hercules Saxoniae and Eustachius Rudius, lectured on the same topics, but treated each subject one year in advance of the Extra-Ordinary professors.

In addition to this knowledge of things pertaining to medicine, Harvey was also trained in Padua in Aristotelian philosophy and in the methods of Aristotelian thought. George Raguseus who signed Harvey's doctoral diploma was, in 1602, second professor of Ordinary Philosophy. But he had only been appointed to this, his first academic post, on 20 October 1601, so that his influence on Harvey cannot have been very profound. When Harvey arrived in 1599 the second professor was Cesare Cremonini, the first Francesco Piccolomini. On 23 June 1601, Cremonini was appointed to succeed Piccolomini. It seems quite likely, therefore, that although Harvey was examined by Raguseus he was taught Aristotelian philosophy by Cremonini. Cremonini had been invited to Padua by the *Riformatori* who had heard excellent reports of his teaching in Ferrara, and on 23 September 1590 he was appointed to fill the vacant chair of the great Aristotelian philosopher, Giacomo Zabarella. Cremonini was welcomed with enthusiasm by the whole University; he was immensely popular with the students and enjoyed great renown in his lifetime throughout the learned world. But Cremonini was not a man of much originality of thought. He prided himself on being the faithful interpreter of Aristotle. He believed that truth resided only in the past and refused to pay any attention to newly discovered scientific truth. As is well known, he opposed Galileo and denied that his view of the universe could be true, preferring to remain a resolute defender of Aristotelian cosmology. While Harvey was at Padua, however, the greatest friendship existed between Cremonini and Galileo, for Galileo had not then publicly proclaimed his acceptance of the Copernican hypothesis. In the years that Harvey was there, Cremonini was lecturing on the *Physics* of Aristotle, and possibly on his *De anima* and *De generatione et corruptione*. So closely did he identify himself with Aristotle that he won the nickname of 'Aristoteles redivivus'. There is one reference to Cremonini in Harvey's writings: in *De generatione*, Harvey disagrees with Cremonini's views on innate heat. But it could be that from Cremonini Harvey learnt much of his love for Aristotle.

While Harvey was at Padua, the chair of mathematics was occupied by Galileo.[38] On 26 September 1592, the *Riformatori* invited him to come from Pisa where he was then teaching 'con sua grandessima laude et si puo dir che sia il principal di questa professione'. He remained in Padua until 1610. According to Galileo himself these were the happiest years of his life. But the fact that he was in Padua at the same time as Harvey has given rise to much speculation concerning the relationship between them. There are those who express surprise that Galileo's progressive views, which they think were well known to all the students in Padua, should have had so little influence on Harvey's attitude to science or medicine. A directly contrary view has also been maintained by those who think that in Harvey's method they can recognise Galileo's teaching, for they believe Galileo to have been the father of experimental research. At various times it has been suggested not only that Harvey attended Galileo's lectures, but moreover, that he lived in his house as a private pupil and that he was a close personal friend of the astronomer. It has also been asserted that Galileo's teaching on the astronomy of Copernicus had a profound influence on Harvey's thinking concerning the circular movement of the blood. The records preserved in the University of Padua and Galileo's own writings show that both those who find a direct influence of Galileo on Harvey, and those who express surprise at not finding it, have failed to take into account all the known facts. First, there is no evidence whatsoever to show that Harvey lived with Galileo. In March 1599, Galileo records that he had as his pupil Alessandro, the son of Alfonso II d'Este (X, 72–3). He gives a list of his private pupils, Italians and others, just after 28 June 1601. Among them was Otto Brahe, nephew of Tycho Brahe. Otto was one of the Councillors in 1600 and, therefore, probably an exact contemporary of Harvey. But Harvey's name does not figure in Galileo's list (XIX, 149–58). The subjects which Galileo taught these young men, his pupils, were perspective, fortification, arithmetic, the elements of Euclid, the use of the compass and other mathematical instruments, mechanics, geodesy, the spheres and cosmography. As far as is known, all these pupils were mathematicians, engineers and architects – not physicians. Secondly, while Harvey was in Padua, Galileo was lecturing in the University on the works of Euclid and on the Book of the Spheres. His private work was chiefly concerned with the mechanics of Aristotle and with the designing and perfecting of various mathematical instruments, such as the geometrical and military compass

34

on which he had begun at the end of 1598 (II, 534–5). In 1597, Galileo had published his *Trattato della sferica ovvero Cosmografia* which was entirely devoted to an exposition of the Ptolemaic system. There is no reason to suppose that what he taught in his lectures in Padua differed from the views expressed in this book. His first public pronouncement on the Copernican system was made at the end of 1604, two full years after Harvey had left Padua, and were it not for the fact that in a private letter to Kepler (X, 67–8), written on 4 August 1597, Galileo reveals his knowledge of Copernicus's theory of the movement of the spheres, it would not have been known that as early as this he had begun to think along these lines himself. In this letter Galileo thanks Kepler for sending him his book *Prodromus*. Although he has as yet only had time to read the preface, he will read the book with pleasure for he is entirely in agreement with Kepler on the truth of the Copernican theory and has been for some time ('quod in Copernici sententiam multis abhinc annis venerim, ac ex tali positione multorum etiam naturalium effectuum causae sint a me adinventae, quae dubio procul per communem hypothesim inexplicabiles sunt'). What he has written about this he has not yet dared to make public, frightened by the fate of Copernicus, who, although he has acquired lasting fame in the opinion of some, yet in the eyes of the multitude, so great is the number of the stupid, is held for a laughing-stock. ('Multas conscripsi et rationes et argumentorum in contrarium eversiones, quas tamen in lucem hucusque proferre non sum ausus, fortuna ipsius Copernici, praeceptoris nostri, perterritus, qui, licet sibi apud aliquos immortalem famam paraverit, apud infinitos tamen (tantus enim est stultorum numerus) ridendus et explodendus prodiit' (X, 67–8). (The reason for Galileo's silence on the Copernican theory between 1597 and 1604 is for his biographers to determine, the fact of this silence remains. If Harvey did attend Galileo's lectures, as he might have done out of curiosity, then all he heard was an exposition of the Ptolemaic system, or some discourse on the elements of Euclid or the mechanics of Aristotle. It was not until August 1602 that Galileo first discussed with Fra Paolo Sarpi his ideas on the magnet, and only in the November in that year is there the first reference in his writings to the isochronism of the pendulum. The direct influence of Galileo on Harvey does not exist, and that it does not should cause no surprise. It is very doubtful whether attendance at lectures on mathematics was required of a student who was in Padua only for the last part of his medical career, for it was a discipline that formed part of the preliminary liberal arts course before the study of medicine proper was begun. Harvey makes only one reference to Euclid in his writings and that is a mistake, for he attributes to Euclid the pronouncement of Archimedes, 'Give me a lever and I will move the earth'. There is little evidence that in his study of the mechanics of muscle contraction, Harvey used any other works than those of Fabricius. His references to astronomy and astronomers in *De generatione* are not entirely flattering and from one or two of his remarks in this same book, it can even be questioned as to whether he really believed that the earth went round the sun.

The years which Harvey spent in Padua were peaceful and unperturbed by any political upheaval. There was no outbreak of plague, and the Acts of the German Nation record no events of any particular interest. In April 1600, the Captain of Padua, Leonardo Moecenigo, entered the city with a great procession accompanied by trumpets and drums. On 3 January 1602, the Podestà, Giovanni Baptista Bernardo, died and his body was taken by ship to Venice. He was succeeded on 3 March by Francesco Bernardo, a member of the same family. About this time, a number of the students absented themselves from Padua and went off to other universities, notably to Parma. So the new Podestà made a public proclamation outside the Schools to the sound of trumpets, ordering all those who had departed to return within a month, or suffer the confiscation of all their possessions.

When the time came for Harvey's examination for his doctor's degree, he had first to submit himself, as in Cambridge, to a private examination by the doctors of the Faculty. After that, his two promoters presented him to the Rector and the day was fixed for his public examination. As he was one of those who received a doctorate by authority of the Emperor, his examination had to take place in the house of the Count Palatine, in the presence of the Rector who could interfere if he thought the questions deliberately unfair, and he had to pay to the Rector and the University the fees normally paid to the Sacred College of Physicians and Philosophers. For his illuminated diploma Harvey paid the University's notary half a ducat. When he finally came to leave the University and the city, he had to have a public proclamation to this effect read in the Schools.

NOTES

1. Bodleian Library, MS. Rawlinson, D. 815. See L. M. Payne, *Journal of the History of Medicine*, XII (1957), 158–64.
2. For information on the curriculum at Cambridge, see William T. Costello, S.J., *The Scholastic Curriculum at Early Seventeenth-Century Cambridge*, Cambridge, Mass., 1958; Mark H. Curtis, *Oxford and Cambridge in Transition*, Oxford 1959.
3. Provision was made for the study of similar subjects at Padua as part of the liberal arts course which the students had to follow before proceeding to the specialised study of medicine or philosophy or both. Between 1593 and 1604, in the lectures on the Humanities, the following texts were read: Aristotle's *Rhetoric* and the Greek Epigrams; Cicero's *Topics* and Sophocles's *Oedipus Tyrannus*; Cicero's *Quaestiones Tusculanarum, In somnium Scipionis*, and some work of Demosthenes; Aristotle's *Poetics;* the first book of the *Odes* of Horace; Livy. The books prescribed for the lectures on logic were those of Aristotle's *Posterior Analytics*. In the course on the moral philosophy of Aristotle, his *Ethics* were read, and once, his *Politics*. It will be noticed that the writings of Plato do not figure in the list.
4. Disputations in which the students took part also occurred regularly in Padua. They were considered a means of teaching the student how to use the knowledge he had acquired: 'Non solum ad veritatis notitiam disputationes conserunt, sed etiam ad exercitationem et rerum quas discimus promptitudinem et solertiam acquirendam et scholarium audaciam in formandam maxime pertinet.' Every doctor reading in arts or medicine was required to hold a public disputation at least twice a year, once before and once after Easter. If he failed to do so, he was liable to a fine of 50 *li.*, of which one third was payable to the Rector, the University, and the Doge, respectively. In every disputation with the students, seven were to take part, of whom the first was to be of the Nation of the Rector, and the seventh a citizen of Padua. While the disputation was in progress, no lectures were to be given. Any student wishing to dispute in medicine had to be of at least two and a half years' standing. More details concering these disputations will be found in the *Statuta Universitatis Artistarum*, published in Venice in 1589. The greater part of the regulations there contained date from 1465, but seem to have been still in force at the end of the sixteenth century. Certain later additions are also contained in the book. For instance, in 1496, it was decreed that any student wishing to dispute publicly in the Schools was to give the Rector a pair of gloves worth 20s., and the Sapiens a pair worth 10s., in addition to certain other charges.

   Provision was also made in Padua for informal disputations in the evenings. They were known as *disputationes circulares* and took place in the *apothecae* and not in the Schools. (Evening disputations of this kind also occurred in the University of Paris.) Between the commencement of the academic year and Easter, every doctor reading in philosophy and medicine was bound, on pain of a fine of 20s. (and no valid excuses except illness), to attend these disputations for at least one hour each day, and there discuss what they had said in their lectures and listen to the students 'benigne et quiete', and resolve their doubts, and everything to be done without abuse or altercation. (A similar clause in the Laudian Statutes at

37

Oxford provided that the lecturer should remain behind after his lecture to resolve the doubts of the students.) If a lecturer wished to change his conclusions from what he had said in his lecture, he could do it here in these evening disputations, provided that he gave notice to the students by the bedellus that he was about to do so. Any student who wished to propose an alternative conclusion might do so, provided that he gave notice of it at least in the morning of the same day, or preferably on the night before, and his proposal would then be discussed. The Rector had to preside over the circle of the medical students and his deputy over that of the philosophers, and they had to note which doctors were absent and see that everything was conducted in a quiet and orderly manner.

5. Sir Geoffrey Keynes, *The Life of William Harvey*, Oxford 1966, p. 15.

6. *Ibid.*, p. 11, *n.* 1.

7. *Ibid.*, pp. 17–18.

8. A. Andrich, *De natione anglica*, 1892, contains a list of the Councillors of the English Nation taken from the University Archives. Two entries for 1600–01 and 1601–02 read 'D. Gulielmus Ameius, Anglus.' Sir D'Arcy Power, *William Harvey*, 1897, pp. 18–20, caused this reading to be verified and confirmed the belief that the surname was a copyist's mistake for *Arveius*. The presence of two stemmata bearing the name *Gulielmus Harveius Anglus* in the courtyard of the University, support this conclusion. All details concerning the Councillors of the English and Scottish Nations in the following paragraphs derive from Andrich's book.

9. *Statuta Universitatis Artistarum*, Venice 1589.

10. His diploma is in the British Museum, MS Sloane 3450.

11. Archivio antico della Università di Padova, MS 465, Matricola della Nazione Germanica Artista, ff. 57 *et seq.*

12. Strangely enough one of the signatories of the German register during this period (13 October 1599) was an Englishman, James Gomond of Kenchester in Hereford-shire. He is described there as φιλιατρος, 'a lover of the art of medicine'. He was probably not a student but a visitor who made a donation to the University and signed the book out of courtesy, *ex more Patavinae Academiae*. There are a number of other instances, though mostly of a later date, in which the matriculation register seems to have served as a 'Visitors' Book'.

13. *Statuta*, I, 3.

14. Archivio del Stato, Studio patavino, Busta n. 192.

15. *Notes to accompany a Facsimile Reproduction of the Diploma . . .*, with a translation by J. F. Payne, M.D., F.R.C.P., London, privately printed at the Chiswick Press, 1908.

16. The Sacred College of Philosophers and Physicians of Padua was a select body within the University. It exercised an authority somewhat similar to that of the College of Physicians of London. It examined candidates for degrees in philosophy and medicine and surgery; it licensed surgeons to practise their craft and it warred with empirics. It was governed by a President, a Syndic, Councillors and a Procurator. It was the President who *ex officio* presided at all examinations, while the jury was composed of professors of the faculty. Between 1598 and 1602 it seems to have had about thirty-one members. Applications for admission to the

College (*aggregazione*) had to be supported by documents to prove that the candidate was the legitimate son of his father, born in legitimate wedlock, that for the last fifty years his family had paid its taxes to the city of Padua and supported itself on its own income, and lastly, that neither he nor his ancestors had ever exercised any mechanical art or been a pedagogue. The election of Fabricius ab Aquapendente, a surgeon, to this body was therefore a considerable event.

17. Jacobus Facciolatus, *Fasti Gymnasii Patavini*, Padua 1757, p. 222.

18. Matthew Lister left Padua without taking a degree and matriculated in the University of Basel in October 1604. On the following 7 November he received a doctorate of medicine in that University. In 1607 he was admitted a Fellow of the College of Physicians in London. He became physician to Queen Anne of Denmark, and later to Charles I. He was knighted in 1636 and died in 1656. Peter Mounsel also visited Basel, presumably on his way back to London, for he signed the register of the Rector in 1605 and subscribed 16s. to the funds. In that year he was appointed professor of Physic at Gresham College, an office which he held until his death in October 1615. Simon Fox, the son of the martyrologist, succeeded Harvey as Treasurer of the College of Physicians in 1629 and was President of the College 1634–40. He died in 1642. Robert Darcey was perhaps the son-in-law to Dr Argent, and son to the 'noble Knight Baronet, Sir Robert Darcie', the post-mortem condition of whose heart Harvey describes in his Second Letter to Riolan. Richard Willoughby may be the same man as the 'Robert Willobe' who was Councillor for the English Nation in 1603. I have not identified Antony Fortescue.

19. Thomas Hearne had received his degree on 19 March 1602 at a similar ceremony in the presence of Count Sigismund. The same Englishmen were present, including Harvey in the rôle of Councillor, and with the addition of an Edward Silyard who has not been identified. Minadous again bestowed the doctoral insignia. Hearne's doctorate, however, was in medicine alone, and instead of Casserius the examiner in surgery was Francesco Mandello. I have found no other reference to him. In addition to Fabricius, Minadous and Raguseus, Hearne's diploma was also signed by Prosper Alpini. He had been appointed to the lectureship on simples in April 1594, with the obligation to read Dioscorides and Galen. He did not have charge of the Orto Botanico until 1603.

20. On his appointment in 1540, Vesalius was described by the Doge as having 'tanta peritia nella anatomia et arte di seccare li corpi humani che l'artificio suo in cio è estimato admirabile', and no less skilled in all the other branches of surgery. This and other references to the dates of appointment of the various professors at Padua derive from the original registers in the Archivio di Stato. Later copies of some of the entries are kept in the University Archives.

21. The reference to 'forty years' seems to imply that Fabricius was already teaching in Padua in 1561, that is for some four years before his official appointment and while Falloppius was still alive. As we know that Vesalius also taught for at least a year if not more before being officially appointed by decree of the Doge, it is safe to assume that the inference is correct. Fabricius took his doctorate in Padua in 1559 and presumably stayed to assist Falloppius.

22. For details of the Anatomical Theatre, see Howard B. Adelmann, *The Embryological*

Treatises of Hieronymus Fabricius of Aquapendente, New York 1942, pp. 8–11; E. Ashworth Underwood, 'The Early Teaching of Anatomy at Padua, with special reference to a model of the Paduan anatomical Theatre', *Annals of Science*, XIX (1963), 1–26.

23. Facciolatus, *Fasti*, pp. 208–09.
24. *Acta nationis Germanicae artistarum et medicorum*. Two volumes, from 1553 to 1616, were editied and published 1911–12 by Antonio Favaro under the title *Atti della Nazione Germanica Artista nello Studio di Padova*. A third volume, 1616–36, edited by L. Rossetti was published by the University of Padua in 1967. The work is continuing, and will be complete in six volumes. For further information on Fabricius's teaching see Giuseppe Favaro, *L'insegnamento anatomico di Girolamo Fabrici d'Acquapendente*, 1921, and Adelmann, *op. cit.* pp. 6–35.
25. *De generatione animalium*, London 1651, p. 19; Willis tr. p. 194.
26. Much information on this subject may be had from Adelmann's edition of *The Embryological Treatises* of Fabricius.
27. See K. J. Franklin, *De venarum ostiolis, 1603, of Hieronymus Fabricius of Aquapendente (1533?–1619)*, Illinois and Maryland 1933.
28. Caspar Bauhin, *De corporis humani partibus externis tractatus*, Basel 1588, Praefatio.
29. Caspar Bauhin, *De corporis humani fabrica, Libri IIII*, Basel 1590, lib. 2, cap. 50.
30. *Ibid.*
31. *Anatomical Lectures*, p. 135.
32. The Latin word is *ira* which is freqently translated as 'wrath', but after Classical times the word seems to have undergone an extension of meaning and to imply more generally 'passion' or 'strong emotion'. Cf. Old French, *irié*, which frequently means 'chagrined'. On the heart as the seat of the emotions, see Index.
33. *De respiratione*, cap. 8, *in fine*.
34. The Acts of the German Nation record anatomies by Casserius in 1585–6, 1594–5, 1595–6, 1597–8, 1604, 1612–13.
35. *Anatomical Lectures*, p. 219. Casserius discovered the adductor hallucis which Harvey calls 'the muscle of Casserius', *Ibid.*, p. 479.
36. According to the Acts, the German Nation presented him with two silver candelabra for this remarkable anatomy.
37. Padua, Museo Civico, B.P. 147.
38. For an account of Galileo at Padua, see Antonio Favaro, 'Diario del Soggiorno di Galileo a Padova, 1592–1610', in *Memorie e documenti per la storia della Università di Padova*, I, Padova 1922. It is included in the volume entitled *Galileo Galilei a Padova. Ricerche e scoperte, insegnamento e scolari*, a collection of the works of A. Favaro, reprinted at Padua, 1968. Also reprinted at Padua in 1966 in 2 vols is A. Favaro, *Galileo Galilei e lo Studio di Padova*, originally published at Florence in 1883.
The references to the works of Galileo are to the National Edition.

Chapter Two

The Discoveries of Realdus Columbus
and their Importance for Harvey

O NE of the great problems which exercised the anatomists of the
second half of the sixteenth century was to explain how the blood
got from the right ventricle of the heart into the left. Though the problem was a simple physiological one and its solution was to be found
by observation and experiment, it was complicated for the sixteenth
century because of its philosophical and theological connotations.
Consequently, any deviation from the received physiological opinion
entailed a modification in philosophical explanation, and thereby the
acceptance of newly-discovered fact was rendered doubly difficult.

As is well known, Galen taught that the blood was formed in the
liver. After the raw aliment had been concocted in the stomach, the
refined portion, or chyle, was conveyed through the portal vein into
the liver where it underwent a further concoction and, freed of im-
purities, became venous blood. At the same time this blood was imbued
with the spirit which gives life and is innate in all living things, that is,
with natural spirit, and hence with the power of itself conveying life
and nourishment. From the liver, this venous blood was transported
through the veins, which originated from the liver, to all the parts of the
body for their nourishment. The different parts used up the nutriment
conveyed to them. According to Galen, each part attracted and retained
only enough blood for its immediate requirements and fresh supplies
of this sufficiency were continually brought to it from the liver. Other
writers seem to have envisaged this as a continuous movement of ebb
and flow in the veins, the blood returning to the liver for fresh supplies
of natural spirit as this was used up by the parts. The movement

occurring in the portal vein was even more complicated. Here it was imagined that two contrary movements occurred, one of chyle going from the stomach to the liver, the other of venous blood returning from the liver to the stomach and ebbing and flowing as the supplies of nutriment which it conveyed to the stomach for its activity were endlessly exhausted. From the liver, the vena cava brought the venous blood to the right ventricle of the heart. (Before it reached the heart, the vena cava gave off a branch, the coronary vein, which supplied the heart itself with natural spirit and nutriment.) From the right ventricle, some of the venous blood was expelled through the pulmonary artery (which was called the arterial vein) into the lungs for their nourishment. The remainder of the venous blood passed through the porosities in the interventricular septum into the left ventricle. The basic principle of life, the spirit or *pneuma*, was held by Galen to exist in the air. It was drawn into the body by the act of inspiration, and passed through the trachea into the lungs, where it was communicated through the ends of the bronchioles into the ends of the pulmonary vein (which was called the venous artery). From the pulmonary vein, the air entered the left ventricle of the heart. There it met the venous blood which had come through the septum, and by means of the innate heat of the heart they were together concocted into vital spirit; that is to say, the venous blood was concocted into arterial blood in which the vital spirit inhered in a manner difficult to explain. The receiving into itself of blood and air, and the driving out of blood, venous and arterial, coincided with the movements of the heart. When the heart was in diastole, it attracted venous blood into the right ventricle and air into the left. It was held to be in diastole when the apex was seen to be drawn upwards towards the base by the action of the straight fibres, with the result that at this moment it presented a rounded appearance because the transverse fibres were then relaxed. Conversely, when the heart was in systole, then it was narrowed by the constricting action of the transverse fibres, and as the straight fibres were then relaxed, the heart was lengthened and the apex of the heart further removed from the base. When the heart was contracted in this manner, blood was expelled from the right ventricle into the pulmonary artery, and from the left ventricle vital or arterial blood was driven through the aorta into the body at large. All the arteries of the body were held to originate from the heart. Some part of the arterial blood, however, did not go out through the aorta but back through the pulmonary vein into the lungs to supply them with vital spirit and arterial blood so that they could live. At the same time, the fuliginous vapours which were the excrement of the concoction in the left ventricle (that every concoction occurring in the body left a residual excrement was axiomatic) were driven back through the same pulmonary vein into the lungs and so breathed out of the body. The movement that went on in the pulmonary vein was, therefore, envisaged as similar to that which occurred in the portal vein: air moved from the lungs to the heart when the heart was in diastole; when it was in systole, fuliginous vapours as well as and distinct from arterial blood were driven back from the left ventricle into the lungs. Moreover, this arterial blood, like the venous blood, ebbed and flowed as the supplies of vital spirit which it conveyed to the parts were endlessly used up by these parts that they might continue to live.

To explain the movement of the blood various analogies were used. It was likened to the movement of the tides which perpetually ebbed and flowed. For the Greeks in particular, it seemed analogous to the movement of the sea by Scylla and Charybdis. The tissues of the body were thought to use up the natural and vital spirits inherent in the venous and arterial blood as the fields used up supplies of rain. So in Aristotle we find an adumbration of a circular movement of the blood which has nothing whatever to do with the physiological circulation as described by Harvey: that the rain falling upon the earth returns to the heavens by evaporation. The analogy with the alchemical processes of distillation was inescapable. So, occasionally, the very word 'circulation' came to be applied to the blood's movement before Harvey, thereby constituting a trap for the unwary who fail to realise the difference between the alchemical and physiological meanings of the word. Most commonly, the analogy applied to the veins and arteries was that of rivers. As the rivers bring life-giving water to the fields, so do the vessels of the body supply the parts. So Shakespeare, in *Coriolanus*, Act I, scene I, sums up in effect the Galenic notions on venous blood when he has the belly say to the rebellious members:

> True is it, my incorporate friends, quoth he,
> That I receive the general food at first,
> Which you do live upon: and fit it is;
> Because I am the store-house and the shop
> Of the whole body: but if you do remember,
> I send it through the rivers of your blood,

> Even to the court, the heart, to the seat o' the brain;
> And through the cranks and offices of man,
> The strongest nerves, and small inferior veins,
> From me receive that natural competency
> Whereby they live . . . .

The fact that in rivers the water does not ebb and flow did not prevent this analogy from becoming part of the common-place notions of the sixteenth and seventeenth centuries. The four great vessels leaving the heart were likened again and again to the four great rivers of Paradise. The rivers, as one early seventeenth-century writer put it, were 'the cherishing veines of the body of every countrey, Kingdome and Nation'. So ingrained was this analogy that even after Harvey's discovery, Sir William Petty, writing of the activities of the merchants of his day, held that they yielded of themselves 'no fruit at all, otherwise than as veines and arteries, to distribute back and forth the blood and nutritive juyces of the Body Politic, namely the product of Husbandry and Manufactures.'

Various difficulties in the Galenic account of the heart's action and the blood's movement become apparent on closer scrutiny. Though the heart's action could be satisfactorily explained as consisting in alternate movements of dilatation and contraction, with or without a moment of quiescence between the two, to decide which was which, while watching a heart beat, was a matter of great difficulty. By the sixteenth century, the different kinds of fibres in the heart were recognised, but to analyse the movement in terms of relaxation and contraction of the various sets of fibres was no mean task. Consequently, there are almost as many opinions in detail as there are anatomists, though a general measure of over-all agreement can be found. To generalise, it may be said that the common opinion was the reverse of the truth, for it was thought that the filling of the heart caused it to strike the chest wall. (It is, of course, while it is emptying that the heart twists and the apex rises and strikes the chest wall.) Some anatomists, following Hippocrates, believed the heart to be a very strong muscle and saw its movement as essentially similar to that of all muscle. Others denied this belief. Why it moved was ascribed to its 'pulsific quality', which are for us words without meaning. Why the blood entered the heart could have diverse explanations, from the 'attractive' power of the heart by which it sucked the blood in, to the belief in Nature's abhorrence of a vacuum. The pulse of the arteries, according to Galen, was due to the contraction of the arterial wall and, also in his belief, was synchronous with the contraction of the heart. Moreover, it must not be forgotten that though we talk of the pulmonary vein as that which enters the left ventricle, and the pulmonary artery as that which leaves the right, before Harvey's discovery of the circulation of the blood these terms were conversely applied. The pulmonary artery was called the arterial vein, and the pulmonary vein the venous artery. Both vessels were held to partake of a dual nature, part vein, part artery, according to the texture of their coats and the offices or functions which they were deemed to perform. Because the 'arterial vein' carried venous blood to the lungs, it was a vein, yet it pulsated like an artery. The 'venous artery' was an artery because it brought air to the heart, yet it did not pulsate. And here there seems to be a contradiction even in Galen's work. In his treatise *On the anatomy of veins and arteries*, he refuted the belief advanced by Erasistratus that the arteries contained air; one might have expected to find him denying that the 'venous artery' contained air. The debate on the content of the pulmonary vein was of long duration. Another problem was presented by the valves of the heart whose existence was known, but whose competence was disregarded. Last, and by no means least important of the difficulties, was the belief that respiration was an action intimately connected with the movement of the heart and, in fact, served the same purpose. The individual points here summarised will become clearer in what follows.

Galen's description of how the blood passed from the right to the left ventricle of the heart will be found in his treatise *On natural faculties*, III, 15, and is as follows:

> in the heart itself, the thinnest portion of the blood is drawn from the right ventricle into the left, for the septum between them has small holes which for the most part can be seen like fossae with wide mouths and they get narrower and narrower as they proceed. It is not possible, however, to see their extreme terminations both because of their smallness and because when the animal is dead, all its parts are chilled and shrunken.[1]

As far as is known, all anatomists writing before Vesalius, apart from Nicholas Massa, concurred in the belief in the existence of the intra-ventricular pores, though many stressed the fact that they could not find them. Massa, in his *Liber introductorius anatomiae*, published in Venice in 1536, denied their existence, saying that the septum was thick and dense. At the same time, however, he proclaimed the existence of a passage which he had found at the base of the heart (presumably a patent foramen ovale). Through this he thought the blood could pass and he further complicated matters by equating this 'cavity' with the third ventricle which Aristotle had described.

When in 1543 Vesalius published his *De humani corporis fabrica*, he made it quite clear that he could not find any pores that penetrated through the septum, but this fact did not lead him in this book to deny their existence:

> The septum of the ventricles, therefore, is, as I have said, made out of the thickest substance of the heart and on both sides is plentifully supplied with small pits (*foveis*) which occasion its presenting an uneven surface towards the ventricles. Of these pits not one (at least in so far as is perceptible to the senses) penetrates from the right ventricle to the left, so that we are greatly forced to wonder at the skill (*industriam*) of the Artificer of all things by which the blood sweats through passages that are invisible to sight from the right ventricle to the left.
>
> (Bk VI, cap. 11, p. 589)

When he revised this passage for the second edition of the *Fabrica*, published in 1555, his doubts had increased:

> Nevertheless, howsoever conspicuous these pits may be, not one of them, in so far as is perceptible to the senses, penetrates through the ventricular septum from the right to the left ventricle. Indeed, I have never come upon even the most obscure passages by which the septum of the heart is traversed, albeit that these passages are recounted in detail by professors of anatomy seeing that they are utterly convinced that the blood is received into the left ventricle from the right. And so it is (how and why I will advise you more plainly elsewhere), that I am not a little in two minds about the office of the heart in this respect.

The reason for Vesalius's hesitation is to be found in his opinion concerning the pulmonary vein. In every description which he gives of this vein, chiefly in Bk III, cap. 15, and Bk VI, caps 12 and 15, both in the 1543 edition and in that of 1555, he states that its use is to bring air from the lungs to the heart and to carry off fuliginous vapours. There is no evidence in either edition of the *Fabrica* to show that Vesalius, great anatomist as he was, saw that this was a Galenic error and that, in fact, the pulmonary vein contained blood. To this point we will return later when considering the work of Columbus. As a result of clinging to this error, Vesalius could find no other means of bringing the blood from the right to the left ventricle except through the invisible pores which he could not find in the septum. Concerning the pulmonary artery also, Vesalius was content with the Galenic view, that it carried blood which had been refined and prepared in the right ventricle of the heart to the lungs for their nourishment. As the thick blood leaving the liver was considered unsuitable nourishment for the light and frothy lungs, which were continually in movement, it was thought that in the right ventricle it underwent a process by which it was rendered fine and thin. (This had the double advantage of making it suitable for the lungs and allowing it more easily to pass through the pores of the interventricular septum.) It was, therefore, also believed that the right ventricle was designed for the express use of the lungs, and those animals which lacked lungs and had hearts with only one ventricle were thought to have a left ventricle only. This view Vesalius expresses in Bk VI, cap. 15, p. 596, in a passage whose wording remained unchanged in the 1555 edition:

> This ventricle indeed, in those animals which possess it, attracts the great force of blood from the vena cava whenever the heart is dilated and distended, and this blood it concocts, the small pits in the ventricle assisting in the process, and refining it by its heat and making it lighter so that it may thereafter be the more fit to be carried headlong through the arteries, it allows the greater part of it to sweat through the pores of the interventricular septum of the heart into the left ventricle; the remainder of the blood, it turns out through the pulmonary artery into the lung while the heart is contracting and compressing itself . . . .

A little further on in the same chapter (p. 598), Vesalius describes the left ventricle and writes:

> Just as the right ventricle attracts the blood from the vena cava, so does the left, when the heart is dilated, draw to itself the air which has been attracted from the lung into the pulmonary vein, and it uses this air to cool its innate heat, to nourish its own substance and to make the vital spirit, so concocting and preparing this air to the end that, together with the blood which has copiously sweated through the ventricular septum from the right to the left ventricle, it may be dispatched into the great artery and indeed into the whole body.

The only alteration which Vesalius made here in 1555 was to change 'the blood which has copiously sweated through' into 'the blood which is thought (*putatur*) to sweat abundantly through'. Vesalius's only contribution, therefore, to this part of the problem of the blood's

47

movement was to cast serious doubt on the existence of the pores in the septum. His promise to advise the reader more plainly elsewhere on his views does not appear to have been fulfilled. In 1555, he apparently had no idea that the hypothesis that the blood passed from the right ventricle of the heart to the left by way of the lungs was true, and he may even not have been aware of the existence of such an hypothesis.

Much has been written about the discovery of the pulmonary transit of the blood. The facts are simple enough; their interpretation somewhat more difficult. The facts are these. In 1553, two years before the revised edition of the *Fabrica* of Vesalius, Michael Servetus published in his theological treatise *Christianismi restitutio*, what appears to be the first account of the pulmonary tranist to appear in the West. (I am deliberately omitting all reference to Ibn an-Nafis, for there is still no proof that his work was known either to Servetus, or Valverde or Columbus.) In 1556, it was described by the Spaniard Juan Valverde da Hamusco in his anatomical textbook *De la composicion del cuerpo humano* and its discovery attributed to Realdus Columbus, his master, whose experiments to prove that blood and not air was contained in the pulmonary vein Valverde described. In 1559, Columbus's own account of the phenomenon and of his experiments was printed in his own book *De re anatomica*. This book was a posthumous publication and, in spite of the date on the title-page, did not appear until early in 1560. Columbus died some time during the summer months of 1559. Neither Valverde nor Columbus makes any reference to the work of Servetus. As Servetus was burnt at the stake in Geneva for heresy on 27 October 1553, he could have had no knowledge of the published works of the Roman anatomists.

From the dates of publication of the three works it would seem obvious that credit for the discovery should go to Servetus. But certain difficulties militate against this assumption. To discuss this problem is, however, outside the scope of this book. A commonly accepted view, at the present time, is that both Servetus and Columbus formulated the hypothesis independently. Though not an impossible conclusion, I think it an unlikely one. However, as Harvey never alludes to the work of Servetus and used only that of Columbus, it is not important for the understanding of his work to decide this question of priority. There is no evidence in the writings of the anatomists of the second half of the sixteenth and early seventeenth century that the work of Servetus was known to them. The first known reference to his *Christianismi restitutio* occurs nearly forty years after Harvey's death, in the *Reflections upon Ancient and Modern Learning* published by William Wotton in London in 1694. Instead, all the anatomists of the period refer to Columbus as the innovator, and it was Columbus's book that Harvey read and used.

It is impossible to say when Harvey first read the writings of Columbus. The knowledge of the pulmonary transit of the blood was, however, one of the necessary pieces of evidence which he had to possess before he could begin to solve the problem of the blood's movement throughout the body. That he knew of it by 1616 is evident because he copied passages from the edition of Columbus's *De re anatomica* printed in 1593 into the notes for the Lectures on the Whole of Anatomy which he delivered to the College of Physicians in London that April. From what has been said in the preceding chapter, it would seem that Fabricius taught the orthodox Galenic view on the movement of the blood, and whether Columbus's views were discussed in Padua even unofficially, is a matter for conjecture. It is, therefore, important not only to examine in detail precisely what Columbus has to say on the subject, but also to decide from the writings of other anatomists to what extent his views were accepted as fact, before Harvey convinced himself of their truth. As well as the knowledge of the pulmonary transit of the blood, Harvey owed to Columbus the correct understanding of systole and diastole of the heart. Each of these subjects will be dealt with in turn.

Columbus's description of the pulmonary transit of the blood occurs briefly in Bk VII of his *De re anatomica*, that is, in the section devoted to the heart and arteries.

There are two cavities in the heart, that is two ventricles not three as it seemed to Aristotle. One of these is on the right, the other on the left. The right ventricle is much larger than the left.[2] In the right ventricle is natural blood, in the left vital. And this is a thing most beautiful in the beholding, the substance of the heart surrounding the right ventricle is rather thin, but surrounding the left is thick, and this is partly for the sake of equilibrium and partly to prevent the vital blood which is very fine from sweating through to the outside. Between these ventricles is the septum, through which nearly everyone thinks that there is a way open for the blood to pass from the right ventricle to the left, and that this may be more easily accomplished they think that it is refined in the transit to be made ready for the generation from it of the vital spirit. But they err by a long way, for the blood is carried to the lung through the pulmonary artery and in the lung it is refined, and then together with the air it is brought through the pulmonary vein to the left ventricle of the heart. This up to now no one has either observed or recorded in writing, although it was most meet to be observed by all.

(Venice 1559, p. 177)

When he reaches the description of the four great vessels of the heart, he says of the pulmonary artery (p. 178):

This enters the lung to bring it blood wherewith it may be nourished and to allow this blood to suffer an alteration for the use of the heart. This pulmonary artery of which we are speaking is of considerable size, truly much bigger than were necessary if its only use were to convey blood from the heart to the lungs over so short a distance.

Having accounted for the name of the pulmonary vein, the 'venous artery', and mentioned its distribution through the lung, he continues (p. 178):

The Anatomists, little prudent in this matter (saving their grace), write of these veins that their use is to carry the altered air from the lungs which like a fan make a breeze around the heart and cool it and not the brain as Aristotle thought. They think the lungs receive I know not what 'capinosous' fumes (for so they call them in their ignorance of language) arising from the left ventricle. This falsehood could not even be spoken were it not that it finds favour with those who, forsooth, believe for certain that the things that are wont to happen in furnaces also occur in the heart, as if in the heart there were green wood which gives off smoke while it burns. Thus far of the use of these veins according to the opinions of other Anatomists. I, indeed, take an exactly opposite point of view, namely, that the pulmonary vein was made to bring blood mixed with air from the lungs to the left ventricle of the heart. This is so true that it is one of the truest things, for if you inspect not only cadavers but also living animals, you will find in all of them that this vein is full of blood, which in no circumstances would be the case if it were constructed solely for the conveying of air and vapours.

The experiment by which he proved that blood was to be found in the pulmonary vein, Columbus describes in Bk XIV, the book he devotes to vivisection (p. 261):

Again, in the fourth [living] dog, you will open the pulmonary vein as far from the heart as possible that you may know for certain whether blood or air is contained in it.

This simple experiment was of such crucial importance for Columbus in the working out of his hypothesis that the blood went through the lungs, that it is of interest to read the fuller account of it as given by Valverde (Bk VI, cap. 14, p. 131^v):

> The office of this vein and artery, according to everyone who has written before me, is of the artery merely to nourish the lung, and of the vein to bring the air from the lung to the left ventricle of the heart, it appearing to them that there could not in any wise be blood in this vein. But, had they made an experiment to prove this (as I have done many times with Realdus, both in living and dead animals), they would have found that this vein is no less full of blood than the other artery. And it cannot be said that the blood enters it after the man is dead, because, when a living animal is opened, so much blood is spilt in the cutting that the heart retains what it holds without letting any of it get out. And if it does get out, it is more reasonable to suppose that it escapes through the mouth of the aorta, through which it goes in ordinary circumstances, than through any other part, Moreover, if it is possible to open the heart suddenly and take all the blood out of it, and then look in this vein, without any doubt it will be found full of blood. This being so, that there is blood in this vein, and that it cannot get there from the left ventricle (as is proved by the position of the valves which we have said are in the mouth of the pulmonary vein), I believe for sure that the blood sweats through from the pulmonary artery into the substance of the lung, where it is rendered more subtle and prepared to be able more easily to be converted into spirit. And then it is mixed with the air which enters through the branches of the trachea, and together with it goes to the pulmonary vein and from thence into the left ventricle of the heart. . . . This is my opinion and it is confirmed by observation, for, having supposed that in the pulmonary vein blood is to be found (as anyone can see for himself if he does not want to believe my statement), it must be said that from there it goes into the left ventricle.

Of equally vital importance was Columbus's realisation of the competence of the valves of the heart, to which Valverde alludes, and the understanding of the precise implication of this phenomenon. In this realisation, the true greatness of Columbus is revealed. He describes the valves as follows, in Bk VII, p. 179:

> In the orifice of the four vessels which are at the base of the heart, eleven membranes are to be observed, of which some are called trisulcate or tricuspid. I say that there are three at the opening of the vena cava, three again at the pulmonary artery, three at the aorta and two at the

pulmonary vein. And their shape is not identical. These which are at the vena cava and pulmonary vein are different in shape from the membranes of the aorta and pulmonary artery, for the former are like three Latin Cs, the latter like arrows. And their use is most admirable and they themselves. By their help we can learn many things pertaining to the right understanding of the use of the heart and of the lungs. Know that just as their shape is different, so also is their employment. The valves of the aorta and pulmonary artery[3] from their internal position are moved outwards to be useful for the emission of blood; the valves of the other two vessels on the contrary are set from outside inwards, so that they seem to be made for the containing of the enclosed blood. It is, moreover, to be noticed that those valves which open from within outwards are crammed with filaments which are spread out on this side and on that through the ventricles. These filaments are made to contain and strengthen the valves. In this great Aristotle was much deceived, for he thought that the filaments of which I am speaking were nerves, and so it happened that Aristotle left it in writing that the heart was the origin of the nerves and, consequently, of sensation and movement. But to return to the aforesaid four vessels. Two of these are so constructed that they lead inwards into the heart, and this happens while the heart is dilating; the other two lead outwards while the heart is constricting. Therefore, when the heart is dilating, it receives blood from the vena cava into the right ventricle, and from the pulmonary vein prepared blood together with air, as we have said, into the left ventricle. And on this account these membranes are loosened and allow ingress. But while the heart is constricting they are shut, lest what they have taken in should go back along the same paths. At the same time the membranes of the aorta and of the pulmonary artery are opened and yield a passage to the spiritous blood which goes out and is poured into the whole body, and to the natural blood which is conveyed to the lungs. And it always happens thus, when the heart is dilating the valves we mentioned first are opened, the rest are shut. And so you will understand that the blood which has entered into the right ventricle cannot go backwards into the vena cava.

The blood cannot go backwards into the vena cava; it cannot, as Valverde had said for him, go backwards into the pulmonary vein. Blood and blood alone is contained in the pulmonary vein. If air is carried to the heart through this vein, then it is mixed with the blood and somehow contained in it. Again, because blood only is always in the pulmonary vein, no fuliginous vapours can be found in it. If they do exist as a result of concoction in the heart, they must be mixed with blood, but then they cannot leave the heart because the valves at the base of the pulmonary vein prevent the return of blood. Fuliginous vapours are a piece of nonsense. The heat of the heart, however it may act, does not resemble a smouldering fire.

Like Vesalius, Columbus had been bred in Galenic tradition, had practised the craft of a surgeon and was a skilled anatomist, and professor of surgery and anatomy in Padua, Pisa and Rome successively. All the knowledge which he had was also available to Vesalius. But armed with three facts, one, that there are no demonstrable porosities in the ventricular septum, two, that there is only blood in the pulmonary vein, three, that the valves of the heart are competent and therefore vital blood cannot return to the lungs, Columbus realised that Galen's theory was wrong. His pupil Valverde, in 1556, had been partially aware of the truth, as had also Servetus in 1553, but both had compromised with Galenic tradition, to a lesser and greater degree, for both, in spite of asserting the septum to be solid, allow a little blood to seep through into the left ventricle. Servetus retained the notion of fuliginous vapours regurgitating through the pulmonary vein for he had no understanding of the true action of the valves of the heart. This compromise between physiological fact and Galenic theory allowed Servetus in particular to preserve intact the Galenic doctrine of the spirits. Columbus, realising that this doctrine of the spirits could not be accommodated to his new physiological findings, proceeded to modify the doctrine. This he explains when he comes to discuss the part played by the lungs in Bk XI, cap. 2.

Having mentioned the various uses of the lungs, to cool the heart, for respiration for the use of the voice, all traditional, Columbus continues p. 223:

> But those who have written before me know all these uses of the lung. In addition to these, I bring forward another of great moment, which they have not even seen through a glass darkly. This is, indeed, the preparation and, so to speak, the generation of the vital spirits which afterwards are greatly perfected in the heart. For the lung receives the air breathed in through the nostrils and the mouth; indeed by means of the arteria aspera it is carried through the whole of the lung, and the lung indeed mixes that air with the blood which leaves the right ventricle of the heart and arrives through the pulmonary artery. This pulmonary artery is so large that it may well be that it brings blood for some additional purpose, besides the nourishing of the lung. The blood which is driven about as a result of the perpetual movement of the lungs, is rendered fine and mixed

with the air, both of which in this battering together and breaking to pieces are made ready, so that, mixed together, the blood and the air may be taken in through the branches of the pulmonary vein and conveyed through its trunk to the left ventricle of the heart. They are indeed conveyed there so wondrously well mixed and refined, that, in addition, there remains only a small amount of work for the heart to do. After this small further elaboration, as if by the application of the tips of the fingers, the heart is left with the vital spirits themselves so that it may distribute them to all the parts of the body by means of the aorta. I fear that this new use of the lungs, which no Anatomist dreamed of till now, must seem a paradox to the unbelievers and the Aristotelians. Them I beg and implore to look upon the size of the lung which could not endure without vital blood, for there is no single part of the body, however small, which is destitute of it. If the vital spirit is not begotten here in the lungs, by what part could it be transmitted to them except by the aorta? But from the aorta no branch, neither big nor very small, is sent to the lungs. How can vital blood be carried to the lung through the pulmonary artery or pulmonary vein, seeing that neither pulsate? And therefore, honest Reader, as I have said, this pulmonary vein[4] was constructed for the purpose which I have said, namely to bring the prepared blood into the heart itself, not to draw it out from the heart and carry it away. And these things which I have said another reason supports. Physicians infer that blood escapes from the lungs and, moreover, are certain, taught by long experience, not only that it is drawn out by coughing but also that it is brightly coloured, thin and beautiful (*floridus est, tenuis et pulcher*) as they have also been wont to say of the blood in the arteries. Whosoever is willing to consider these reasons with an open mind, will, I know well enough, agree, and will allow a place to be given to the truth, even though Galen, the great philosopher and chief of all physicians, if we except Hippocrates, does in fact seem to have been ignorant of this use of the lungs. Let be, he is a great philosopher and a still greater physician, and yet it is not surprising that these things and many others have been concealed from man. Yet truly, there is a race of men stupid, and ignorant, who have neither the wish nor the ability to find anything new. And therefore, whatever a physician with a great name writes, they immediately subscribe to it, nor will they depart from their beliefs not one jot. But you, honest Reader, a pupil of learned men and most zealous for the truth, I beg of you try the experiment in living animals dissecting them alive, I admonish you, I exhort you, try the experiment I say, and find out whether what I have said agrees with the thing itself. In these creatures you will find that the pulmonary vein is full of that kind of blood [sc. as mentioned above, arterial or vital] and not full of air or fumes, sooty fumes as they call them, may it please God! and there the pulse simply does not exist. For the pulse arises from the heart, just as great Galen abundantly proved in his book *An sanguis in arteriis contineatur contra Erasistratum.*

Confirmation of his hypothesis that the vital spirit is generated in the lungs and not in the heart, Columbus finds in the coronary vein and artery (p. 177):

> The heart is encircled by the coronary vein that it may be nourished by the blood from this vein. And with this vein is associated the artery also called coronary, and sometimes indeed two. And this that the substance of the heart may be vivified by its power. And for this reason a man may doubt and from these said facts adduce a completely valid argument, as to whether the vital spirits are not generated in the lungs rather than in the heart. However, I leave the discussing of difficulties of this kind to the great philosophers. It will be enough for me, I think, if, as far as in me is possible, I describe correctly the parts of the body and their uses.

Columbus's account of the pulmonary transit of the blood reveals the anatomist and physiologist reasoning from observed phenomena. The septum is a solid wall, therefore no blood goes through. The size of the pulmonary artery suggests that it conveys more blood than is necessary merely for the nurturing of the lungs, and so supports the hypothesis that by this route the blood reaches first the lungs, then the pulmonary vein and lastly the left ventricle. Experiments prove that only blood is contained in the pulmonary vein. The valves of the heart are competent, therefore nothing passes through when they are closed, not even fuliginous vapours, which do not in fact exist because there is no smouldering fire in the heart. The blood enters the right ventricle of the heart from the vena cava and leaves by the pulmonary artery. Blood returns from the lungs by the pulmonary vein into the left ventricle and leaves through the aorta. And that this goes on all the time and in this direction only is proved by the valves of the heart. The only compromise that Columbus made with authority concerned the generation of vital spirits. As, for various reasons, it seemed to him that they could not be made in the heart, then they had to be made in the lungs. Yet from his remarks about leaving difficulties of this kind to philosophers, it may, perhaps, be asked how much he believed in their real existence.

On this point, the opinion of his pupil and colleague, Valverde, is interesting. In 1552, Valverde published in Paris a treatise entitled *De animi et corporis sanitate tuenda*, much of which is concerned with philosophical notions and speculations concerning the soul. The generation of the spirits he there discusses in the following terms (p. 145):

> Since then reasoning is in the mind, the mind in the soul, the soul in the spirit, the spirit in the body and the spirit passes through the veins and arteries, the blood and the nerves, and sets the animal in motion and sustains the dependent mass of the body and bears it around and makes it partake of sensation, the substance of the spirits is the vaporous exhalation of the fine blood, an exhalation which dwells in the ventricles of the brain as in its permanent abode. It is to be asked whether their first origin is in the brain or rather whether, after being generated in the left ventricle of the heart, they are carried to the ventricles of the brain so that there, as being in their proper organ, they may perform their proper function and dispense their virtue from thence into the whole body through the nerves.

This orthodox opinion on the generation of animal and vital spirits, Valverde repeats in his *De composicion del cuerpo humano* of 1556, where, in Bk IV, cap. 1, p. 102, he writes:

> In the heart are generated the spirits of life, called for that reason the vital spirits. The substance of these spirits is the vaporous exhalation of the blood together with some part of the air which we take in continuously through the mouth and nose while breathing.

In spite of this, a few pages later in cap. 7, p. 104ᵛ, when he is describing the uses of the lungs, he says:

> The principal office of the lungs is to receive the air and prepare it so that from it can be made the vital spirits (if indeed they are made). . . .

It is not perhaps unfair to either of them to suggest that this doubt reflects the opinion of Columbus. To retain the notion of their existence was, as has been said, the only compromise with tradition that Columbus made. That he did compromise on this point is not surprising, for it was to be fully another hundred years before men were ready to jettison the notion of vital spirits.

Columbus did not live to hear how his ideas were received after the publication of his book. It does not seem to have had immediately great or widespread repercussions. Galenic theory was too firmly ingrained for novelties to win an easy acceptance. Perhaps the first allusion to his work was made by Falloppius in the public anatomy which he gave at Padua during the winter of 1560-1. On that occasion, he took the opportunity to ridicule the whole idea. Being a convinced Galenist, Falloppius believed that the movement of the heart was due to its 'pulsific faculty', that this movement was the cause of the heat in the heart which in turn bred the vital spirits. He believed in the existence of the pores in the ventricular septum, the entry of air through the pulmonary vein and the regurgitation therein of fuliginous vapours. His main quarrel with Columbus is joined on the issue of the place of generation of vital spirits. 'I am amazed', he says, 'at certain anatomists who say that the vital spirit is generated in the lungs; I do not know where they keep their brains.' And to refute this idea he produces various anatomical arguments, based chiefly on the connections of the vessels in the foetal heart, and on the observation that fish have no lungs, yet they move and therefore have vital spirit, which cannot be generated in the lungs. He does not bother to criticise Columbus's anatomical and experimental findings, for he does not take them seriously.

It has already been said that in 1555, when he published the revised edition of the *Fabrica*, Vesalius did not appear to know anything of the pulmonary transit of the blood. This was not the case when, in December 1561, he wrote his reply to Falloppius's *Observationes anatomicae*. By this date he had read Valverde's textbook with close attention and is liberal in his criticism, even in his abuse. There is, however, nothing to show that he had read Columbus's own book. Though he does not refer to the whole theory of the pulmonary transit of the blood as such, he alludes to one of its fundamental truths:

> And although in the Spanish textbook of Valverde there are many instances from which it is most easy to choose any to show that neither he nor his master Columbus was even slightly read in the text of Galen or of other writers, yet this is revealed in no perfunctory manner in those places in which he boasts that he himself discovered that the pulmonary vein contains blood, seeing that, forsooth, this very matter was so fully and truly investigated by Galen and many others besides.

Why then did Vesalius persist in saying that there was air in the pulmonary vein, particularly as he doubted the existence of the intraventricular pores? There is little doubt that Vesalius's animosity was part, at least, born of spite and offended *amour-propre*. To illustrate the book he published in 1556, Valverde had used copies of Vesalius's pictures, albeit with due acknowledgement and flattering explanation. This act Vesalius could not forgive. He retaliated by calling Valverde one 'who never put his hand to a dissection' and who was totally ignorant even of the first principles of medicine. Though Valverde, quite clearly from his book, was no great anatomist, there is at least some exaggeration in Vesalius's charge. Vesalius's quarrel with Columbus was of even longer standing and is too complicated in the unravelling to detain us here. The basic cause was simple enough. Columbus had dared to criticise Vesalius in public, and the grounds of his criticism were fully justified. It has been unfortunate for Columbus that later writers have valued him at Vesalius's estimation. They remember that Vesalius called him 'ignorant of letters', but forget that in 1540 he was equated with no less a scholar than John Caius, when they were jointly appointed to lecture to the students in Padua on the philosophical texts of Aristotle in the original Greek; they remember that Vesalius damned with faint praise his skill as an anatomist, but forget that Guinther of Andernach referred to him as 'insignis medicinae professor'.[5]

Before 1561 was over, the first approbatory reference to Columbus had appeared in print. It came from Paris in the *Anatomie universelle du corps humain* published in that year by Ambroise Paré, who is thus the first anatomist to take the new theory seriously, although he was not convinced of its truth. When speaking of the heart and lungs, Paré adopts the Galenic view. When he comes to the pulmonary vein and artery, however, after accounting in traditional manner for their respective names, venous artery and arterial vein, he continues (Bk IV, cap. 12):

> Here wee meet with a difficulty, which is, by what way the blood is carried out of the right into the left ventricle. *Galen* thinkes that there be certaine holes in the partition made for that purpose, and verily there are such, but they are not perforated. Wherefore *Columbus* hath found out a new way, which is that the blood is carried to the lungs by the *vena arteriosa*, and there attenuated, and carried from thence together with the aire by the *Arteria venosa* to the left ventricle of the heart; this he writes truely very probably.

Paré it would seem was prepared to adopt Columbus's view without realising that it could not be accommodated with Galenic theory. He did not understand that the essential feature of Columbus's discovery was not so much the true pathway of the blood, as the conviction of the competence of the valves of the heart, a conviction which precluded any compromise with Galen. But in this Paré was not alone. It is not, however, surprising to find that he was thus aware of the newest theories. Such was ever his reputation. Nor is it surprising that he makes no reference to the site of the generation of vital spirits. As a practising surgeon such matters did not concern him deeply.

Another early reference, this time to Valverde's work, occurs in the *De anatomia corporis humani libri VII* of Guido Guidi. Guidi had been appointed professor of Philosophy and Medicine in Pisa by Duke Cosimo I in 1547, while Columbus was still professor of anatomy in that University. (Columbus went to Rome in 1548.) At that time also, Valverde was already working with Columbus so that Guidi may have known both men personally. Although Guidi's book was not published until 1611, edited by his nephew, Guidi had died in Pisa in 1569. Consequently his reference to Valverde's work must fall between 1556 and that year. That he did not know Columbus's own book is evident from the fact that his allusions are only to Valverde's incomplete account of the pulmonary transit of the blood. Despite the description in Valverde's book of the experiment to prove that blood alone is to be found in the pulmonary vein, it is of this that Guidi is not entirely convinced (Bk VI, cap. 4, p. 298):

Ancient writers (Galen, *De usu partium*, VI, c. 17) said that air alone was carried through it, asserting that, if perchance they found any blood in it in dissecting a cadaver, it was not naturally there but was driven into it by some force or other while the beast was dying. More recent writers (Valverde, Bk VI, cap. 14) assert that blood is naturally contained in it, that this can be verified by using one's eyes. Having opened the chest in a living animal and having cut the heart and taken off the blood, they then divided the pulmonary vein itself and they affirm that in it they find blood which they think cannot possibly be expelled into it by the heart. They add that if the heart is forced to expell blood, it would more easily have power to drive it into the aorta. They think that the pulmonary vein drinks blood from the pulmonary artery in the lung and brings this blood to the left ventricle of the heart, for otherwise they see no way by which it can receive blood from the right ventricle. But however things may really happen, it is certain that the pulmonary vein has a single, fine sheath like all other veins and by nature is soft, so that it can quickly and easily take in the air in the lung which is brought through the trachea, and carry it to the heart.

59

Guidi's perplexity is obvious. He believes in Galenic theory, in concoction in the heart, entry of air through the pulmonary vein, regurgitation of fuliginous vapours, and he holds that the contraction of the heart is contemporaneous with the contraction of the arteries (Bk VI, cap. 5, p. 301). It is when he comes to describe the septum of the heart that he reveals how much he is in two minds about the problem. As no pores can be demonstrated going through it from side to side, he is forced to conclude that most of the blood must go, as he has already described, through the pulmonary artery, the lungs and the pulmonary vein to reach the left ventricle, 'although you may say that some portion of it is refined in the right ventricle and passes into the left *per foramina obscura*, through some hidden pores'.

The imperfect account of the pulmonary transit as given by Valverde, rather than that of Columbus, was again adopted later in the century by Carlo Ruini in his *Dell' anotomia et dell' infirmita del cavallo*, published in Bologna in 1598. The book itself is an outstanding achievement both from the point of view of its content and of its illustrations. It is the first systematic account of the anatomy of the horse to have been published. It deals with the subject after the manner of Vesalius, and its illustrations are by no means inferior to those of the *Fabrica*. Ruini's account of the pulmonary transit is not, however, entirely consistent. He denies the existence of ventricular pores and holds that the right ventricle prepares the blood and sends it to the lungs through the pulmonary artery, and that the left ventricle receives back this prepared blood and concocts it into vital spirit. He also explains that the valves of the heart prevent regurgitation:

> L'officio suo è quando il cuore s'allarga, aprendosi, di lasciare entrare li sangue, e li spiriti dall'arteria venale nel ventricolo manco, e interiore, quando si ritira il cuore, che il sangue, e li spiriti non ritornino di nuovo nell'arteria venale.

From this it would seem that he thinks that blood mixed with air returns through the pulmonary vein to the heart. When, however, in the next chapter he describes the office of the pulmonary vein, he writes:

> L'officio . . . dell'arteria venale è di portar l'aere dagli polmoni al ventricolo manco del cuore, e di condur fuori nello stringersi il cuore quelli escrementi fuliginosi, che sono prodotti dalla mutatione dell'aere

attratto nel sinistro ventricolo nell'aprirsi il cuore dal nativo calore;
e di sommostrare ancora alli polmoni sufficiente sangue sottile, e
spiritoso . . .,

thereby contradicting the statement he has already made. It is difficult
to say what he really believed. He does not mention any authorities
for his opinion, and it is possible that, having convinced himself that
the septum was solid, he read and adopted Valverde's account and then
reverted to the Galenic view. In spite of this, there have been some
historians of medicine to hail Ruini as having anticipated Harvey in
the discovery of the circulation of the blood throughout the whole
body. There is no evidence that Harvey knew anything of Ruini's work.

If proof were wanted that Servetus's work was unknown to the
sixteenth-century anatomists, it could well be had from the next
reference to the pulmonary transit of the blood. This is to be found in
the treatise *De medicina veteri et nova* written by Guinther of Andernach
and published from Basel in 1571. Servetus had at one time been his
pupil in Paris, and it is to Servetus that Guinther alludes in the preface
of his edition of Galen's works printed in Basel in 1539, saying that
Servetus frequently helped him with the dissections, for he was a
man distinguished by every literary achievement and second to none
in anatomical knowledge. As Vesalius also assisted Guinther in this task,
this is no mean praise. It would, therefore, not be unreasonable to
suppose that, of all the anatomists of the time, Guinther at least might
have had some knowledge of Servetus's description of the pulmonary
transit of the blood. But this is not the case. The account which Guinther
gives of the phenomenon in this book is based directly on Columbus's
writing. The phenomenon is not criticised but adopted. Guinther's
book takes the form of a series of dialogues between master and pupil,
Geron and Mathetes. When Mathetes asks the use of the pulmonary
vein (Comment. I, Dial. 5, p. 179), Geron replies:

> To bring blood mixed with air from the lungs to the left ventricle, not
> unchanged air to serve as a breeze for the heart like a fan and cool it, as
> some think; but first, in the lungs, the blood is refined and then together
> with the air is brought through the pulmonary vein to the heart.

Still more significant as proof that Guinther understood the basic
essentials of the theory and was convinced of the truth of the hypothesis,
is the fact that Geron is made to express the positive statement that when

the valves of the heart are closed, nothing can pass through them (Ibid., p. 181):

> When the heart is dilated it takes in blood from the vena cava into the right ventricle, and from the pulmonary vein into the left ventricle not only blood that has been elaborated but also mixed with air. And this because the membranes at the base of the vessels sink down and allow a passage to the substance which enters. Now, when the heart contracts, the membranes in the mouth of those vessels are shut, lest what they have taken in should go back by the same route. At the same time the mouths of the aorta and pulmonary artery are opened to yield a passage to the spiritous blood which is distributed throughout the whole body, and to the natural blood which is conveyed to the lungs. In short, when the heart is dilating, the mouths of the first-named vessels are opened, their membranes sunk down, while those of the latter vessels are closed, their membranes being raised up. For this reason, the blood which has entered into the right ventricle of the heart can in no wise go back into the vena cava. . . .

Though this passage reads much like a copy of Columbus's own text, Guinther is not following Columbus in every detail. It is true that he speaks in much the same terms as Columbus of the preparation of the blood in the lungs by its continual battering and its mixing there with the inspired air, but he does not believe that the vital spirits are created in the lungs. Instead, he speaks of the heart as the fount and origin of all the arteries, of the *anima irascibilis*, and of innate heat, the laboratory and abode of the vital spirit. He does not seem to have been troubled as Columbus was by the thought that unless the vital spirits were made in the lungs, the lungs would be deprived of them. Guinther, however, does not envisage the concotive action of the heart in terms of a slow fire and conseqeuntly, there is no reference in his book to fuliginous vapours.

It would seem that the next complete acceptance of Columbus's hypothesis came from the professor of anatomy at Basel, Felix Plater. In his textbook, *De corporis humani structura et usu*, printed in Basel in 1583, he states all the essential features of the theory, including the competence of the valves of the heart. He keeps the generation of vital spirits in the heart, but thinks that the fuliginous vapours are given off in the lungs during the process of preparation which the blood and air there undergo. He makes no reference to either Valverde or Columbus. As in many respects his account of the phenomenon is similar to that given by Guinther of Andernach, it could be that it was from Guinther that Plater derived his knowledge. Seven years later, in 1590, another professor of the University of Basel, Caspar Bauhin, published his anatomical textbook *De corporis humani fabrica Libri IIII*. In this he could not make up his mind which theory to adopt. When speaking of the vessels in the lungs (p. 179), he says that the pulmonary artery brings blood for their nourishment and that the pulmonary vein takes 'arterial blood, or rather external air attracted in through the trachea and prepared in the lungs, to the heart for its cooling and brings back the fuliginous exhalations of the heart to the lungs.' When he writes of the ventricular septum (p. 258), he quotes Galen's opinion and adds:

> Galen wants the pores to go right through the septum so that through them the blood may be carried from the right ventricle into the left and mixed with the spirits; truly its substance is indeed pitted and more particularly on the right (that the blood may be made more subtle), but it does not seem to need pores. Nor would they have been any use, since the blood may be carried through the pulmonary artery to the lungs where, having been rendered more fine, it can then be brought, together with the air, to the left ventricle through the pulmonary vein. If the venous blood can flow so easily through into the left ventricle, why, having been made spiritous and warmer and finer, does it not flow back into the right ventricle through the selfsame pores in the septum and make a confusion in the order of things?

This question was to be asked again many years later by Harvey. But before that, in 1587, it was put in precisley the same words by Julius Caesar Arantius in his *Anatomicae observationes* published in Venice in that year (p. 93). Perhaps Bauhin's own hesitation was increased by reading this chapter, for in it Arantius says that he does not think that either the opinion of the Ancients or that of Columbus is necessarily true, and he asks a series of questions on both sides. The answers he gives to these questions are, in the sight of modern knowledge, inadequate, but convincing for his time. For instance, he answers the objection to the impossibility of contrary motion occurring in the pulmonary vein, by citing the contrary movements of blood and chyle in the portal vein. By 1605, when his anatomical textbook was revised and enlarged and re-issued as the *Theatrum anatomicum*, Bauhin had become still more undecided (p. 422):

> These pores (*spiracula*) are very conspicuous in the heart of an ox after it has been boiled for a long time. However, there are some who deny

63

this passage thinking that through the pulmonary artery the blood is taken from the right ventricle to the lungs. One part of it remains there in the lung for its nutrition; the other undergoes a further alteration in the lungs and, mixed with the air which is attracted hither, is carried through the pulmonary vein to the left ventricle for the generation and nurturing of spirit and vital blood. This opinion, indeed, pleased me at one time. But now we will leave these matters to the philosophers, for our intention is to describe, as far as with God's help we are able, the true structure of the parts and their use.

There is no doubt that what he had seen in that ox's heart shook Bauhin's belief in the truth of Columbus's theory. This ox's heart makes its appearance in many subsequent textbooks of anatomy and even in Harvey's lectures on the Whole of Anatomy in 1616, for it was this *Theatrum anatomicum* of Bauhin that he used as the basis for his own anatomical commentary.

By the end of the sixteenth century, it is clear that Columbus's theory had by no means won any kind of general acceptance. Nor had it provoked any great storm of abuse. In 1586, Archangelo Piccolomini of Ferrara attacked it in his *Anatomicae praelectiones*. He had succeeded Columbus as professor of anatomy at Rome, knew the writings of Valverde and Columbus, but denied that the valves of the heart were competent, holding instead to the old Galenic opinion. Other anatomists with their own opinions were not wanting. In 1565, Leonardo Botallo thought he had found the real explanation of how the blood got from the right to the left ventricle, and in his small tract, *Vena arteriarum nutrix a nullo antea notata*, published from Paris in that year, described the 'vein' which he had found connecting the right and left ventricles. He failed to realise that what he was describing was the abnormal persistence of the foramen ovale. His contemporaries were not so misled, and it was quickly pointed out by Caspar Bauhin and others, that this phenomenon had already been described by Galen and more recently by Vesalius and by Arantius in his *De humano foetu libellus* (Basel 1579). Harvey himself in *De motu cordis*, cap. 6, refers to this 'discovery' of Botallus and characteristically excuses his error on the grounds that the persistence of the foramen ovale is more frequent and of longer duration than is generally supposed, adding:

I do confess that when I myself first found this in a Rat of full growth, that I did imagine some such thing (p. 46).

Other writers to have their own views were Francis Ulm (Umeau) and Constantius Varolius. In 1578, Ulm published a treatise from Paris, *De liene libellus*, in which he rejected the opinion of Columbus chiefly on the grounds that the lungs in the foetus do not concoct vital spirit:

> Nor indeed should we believe Realdus Columbus, a man most certainly learned and in anatomical matters highly experienced, when he says that he has found an obvious way by which the blood can be introduced into the arteries, namely the pulmonary vein. . . .

Ulm had his own views, to the effect that the concoction of the spiritous blood occurred in the spleen and was from thence transferred to the aorta and so to the left ventricle of the heart. But, his contemporaries objected, surely the valves at the base of the aorta prevent this. Varolius in his *De resolutione corporis humani*, published in Frankfurt in 1591, did not believe that any blood went from the right to the left ventricle, but rather that the arteries brought chyle mixed with blood direct to the left ventricle where it was elaborated and mixed with air to form vital spirit. Though references to the opinions of these two writers appear from time to time in the contemporary anatomical textbooks, they are almost always derided. As will be seen later, others with equally ludicrous theories which they firmly espoused were not wanting in the years to come.

No mention has so far been made of Caesalpinus for the reason that there is no proof that his work was known to Harvey until some time after *De motu cordis* was written. It is, moreover, remarkable that few contemporary anatomists refer to the writings of Caesalpinus. It is almost as if they belonged to the domain of philosophical speculation rather than to the practical world of anatomical study and so were neglected by those with more immediately concrete and physical interests. However, since, in 1655, Giovanni Nardi first advanced the claim that Caesalpinus had anticipated Harvey in the discovery of the circulation of the blood throughout the whole body, there have been some critics to give their blessing to this belief. But it is a belief which seems to be more founded on wishful thinking than on the texts of Caesalpinus's books. Indeed, some seem to have fallen into the error against which Sir George Ent so powerfully warned his hearers when he delivered his anatomical lectures before the College of Physicians in London in 1665. They have read into these texts meanings which were not intended by their author, and, as Ent says, by this device it is possible to prove that even Galen knew that the blood circulated throughout the body. To discuss in detail Caesalpinus's writings and the claims made on his behalf is irrelevant for our present purpose. Suffice it to say that he did know of the pulmonary transit of the blood and, perhaps, understood its significance. But in his writings there are a number of other and directly contradictory pronouncements such as:

> In the heart is the fountain of the blood which is distributed into the four veins, namely the vena cava, the aorta, the pulmonary vein and the pulmonary artery, which irrigate the whole body like the four rivers that flow out from Paradise (*Speculum artis medicae Hippocraticum*, Rome 1601, here quoted from Frankfurt 1605, p. 1).

To go beyond this and maintain that Caesalpinus had any clear idea of the direction of venous blood flow throughout the whole body is patently untrue. The whole controversy would seem to have arisen from the fact that when he does describe correctly the manner in which the blood enters and leaves the heart, he uses the word *circulatio*. One such description occurs in his *Questionum peripateticarum libri quinque*, first published in Florence in 1571 (but here quoted from the 1588 edition, col. 528):

> The lung, therefore, drinking the warm blood from the vein like an artery out of the right ventricle of the heart, and giving it up through an anastomosis to the venous artery [*sc.* pulmonary vein] which goes to the left ventricle of the heart, effects the cooling of this blood by means of the cold air which in the meantime has been sent through the channels of the arteria aspera that lie alongside the venous artery, not however using communicating mouths (*osculis*) for this purpose, as Galen thought, but only contact. With this circulation of the blood from the right ventricle through the lungs to the left ventricle of the heart, those things which can be seen in dissections most admirably agree. For there are two vessels which end in the right ventricle and two in the left. Of these two, only one gives a passage inwards, the other only outwards, for the valves are so constituted for that purpose. The vessel which gives entry to the right ventricle is called the vena cava and is a large vein; the vein which leads into the left ventricle from the lung is little and has only one coat like all the other veins. In the left ventricle, the vessel which leads outwards is the great artery, called the aorta; from the right ventricle a little vessel goes towards the lungs and it has a double coat as have all the other arteries.

In this passage, Caesalpinus is not applying the word *circulation* to the movement of the blood in the vessels, but to the action of cooling the hot blood from the heart. He is not calling the 'venous artery' a vein, and the 'vein like an artery' an artery, because of the direction of the flow of blood which they contain, but because he thinks that the different nature of their coats accounts for the different kind of blood present in each. For confirmation that this is indeed his meaning, the following passage from his *Speculum artis medicae Hippocraticum*, Bk VI, cap. 9 (Frankfurt 1605, p. 442), may be quoted:

On the left side there are two lobes of the lung and the same number on the right, and a small third lobe beside the vena cava. The lung takes in the spirit from the outside [*spiritum externum, sc.* external air] and transmits it through the trachea, which is broken up into many branches and disseminated into all the lobes along the vena cava and aorta so that the heat of the heart may be kept within bounds. Galen thought (*De usu partium*, IV, 4) that it was so in order that the animal spirit might be more fully nourished by that [external] spirit. Which opinion Aristotle refuted, saying that the internal fire was not nourished by spirit (*De respiratione*), but that spirit was made by the heating up of humours, by their lifting up and pushing down, whence comes the pulse and respiration. Therefore, hot blood is carried out of the heart from the right ventricle through the artery which Galen calls the arterial vein, into the lung, and is returned again to the heart through the vein which goes out from the left ventricle and which Galen calls the venous artery. Meanwhile, in its passage, the blood is cooled by the cold air which is breathed in to the branches of the arteria aspera which lie beside the veins and arteries, with the result that by a kind of *circulation* the blood is perfected into the nature of spirit, first in the right ventricle and then in the left. And so the vessel leading out from the heart is truly an artery as is seen by its double coat designed to prevent the spirit from evanescing. The vessel leading into the heart is a vein in that it has but a single coat (Galen, *De usu partium*, VI, 10), for it contains blood which has been cooled.

Here it is clear that the word *circulation* is being used of a process which has nothing to do with the physiological circulation described by Harvey. Caesalpinus is not really concerned with the movement of the blood but with the manner of its cooling. And it is on this point that he disagrees with Galen, who believed that the ends of the bronchioles communicated with the ends of the blood vessels in order that the cold air breathed in could have a direct effect on the hot blood. The manner of cooling which Caesalpinus favours is like the alchemical process of heating and cooling known by the technical term of *circulatio* or 'circulation'. It is to this process that he is alluding.

★   ★   ★

The second debt which Harvey owed to Columbus is to his observations on systole and diastole of the heart. To watch the movement of the heart. and to analyse its movement into the terms of systole and diastole was no mean task. Harvey gave eloquent expression to the difficulties in the first chapter of *De motu cordis*:

> When I first gave my mind to vivisections as a means of discovering the motions and uses of the heart, . . . I found the task so truly arduous, so full of difficulties, that I was almost tempted to think, with Fracastorius, that the motion of the heart was only to be comprehended by God. For I could neither rightly perceive at first when the systole and when the diastole took place, nor when and where dilation and contraction occurred by reason of the rapidity of the motion, which in many animals is accomplished in the twinkling of an eye, coming and going like a flash of lightning; so that the systole presented itself to me now from this point, now from that; the diastole the same; and then everything was reversed, the motions occurring, as it seemed, variously and confusedly together.[6]

In the following discussion, we will attempt to set out the various relevant opinions on the manner in which the heart effected its movements, but we will omit all considerations of the reasons given for its movement.

Hippocrates taught that the heart was 'a very strong muscle', and consequently its movement was generally, but not always, thought of in terms of the movement of muscles. That it was a special kind of muscle was taken into account. Aristotle had divided all movement into three categories: voluntary, involuntary and non-voluntary. Galen had taken over these categories and considered them respectively as movement which was subject to the will, contrary to the will, and 'serving the needs of the body'. As these latter occurred in the body without the intervention of the will, either for or against, they were held to be associated with the natural spirit and were therefore known as natural movements. Movements of defaecation and micturition, for example, came into this category. Voluntary movements, on the other hand, were associated with the animal spirit, and chief of these was the movement of muscle and the movement of the joints of the body.

The diversity of these categories proved a source of much heated argument and debate over problems such as the movement of the lungs. The movement of the heart was generally categorised as natural, for although it was a muscle it was not controlled by the will.

When it is realised that the sixteenth and early seventeenth-century anatomists had no real understanding of what was actually involved in the movement of muscle, it is obvious that the statement that the heart moves like a muscle is little more than an empty phrase. They did not know what was the essential contractile element in muscle; they did not know whether contraction or relaxation was its essential movement. Though they might attempt to analyse movement into the terms of alternate contraction and relaxation of different sets of fibres, they did not realise that contraction was of prime importance. Moreover they did not consider diastole of the heart as a passive state, but as active dilatation during which the blood was drawn into its cavities.

With this preliminary we will turn to Vesalius's description in the *Fabrica*, Bk VI, cap. 10, of the manner in which he thinks the heart moves. After saying that as long as an animal lives, its heart is alternately dilated and contracted, with sometimes a moment of quiescence between these movements, he describes the manner in which it is dilated. He says that the dilatation of the heart, that is the pulling up of the tip towards the base and the distending of the sides of the heart, is effected by the action of the straight fibres which contract and pull the tip upwards. In these words he has described an action which does not occur, for in diastole the heart increases in length and in circumference. However, he thinks that this action corresponds to dilatation or enlarging of the internal cavities of the heart, and this he proves to his own statisfaction by the example of a bunch of rushes. If these are tied together into the shape of a pyramid and the tip is pushed towards the base, the space in the centre of the bunch will be seen to be bigger. From this it is quite clear that Vesalius is thinking of diastole as an active movement designed to draw the blood into the heart. Using again the example of the bunch of rushes, he thinks that when the heart constricts, that is to say when the tip recedes from the base, the straight fibres relax and the transverse fibres constrict. As will be seen later, Harvey gave this whole idea short shrift in *De motu cordis*, cap. 2.

A cognate problem was that of the systole and diastole of the arteries. Galen had taught that the contraction of the heart occurred at the same moment as the contraction of the arteries, and that their dilatation was likewise synchronous. Moreover, Galen thought that he had proved by means of a hollow reed inserted into a severed artery, that the arterial pulse was conducted from the heart along the walls of the arteries, that is to say, that it was due to the contraction of the arterial wall.[7] Such in the sixteenth century was the generally accepted theory, or at least, the opinion to which lip-service was paid. As there was no correct knowledge of which was the systole and which the diastole of the heart, the mistake here is easily understandable. The views on the pulse which Vesalius expresses in the *Fabrica* are orthodox and singularly unrevealing, for he does not mention the relation in time of the arterial pulse to the heart, but merely says that the pulse originates from the heart (Bk VI, cap. 15), and that its use and that of respiration are identical (Bk VI, cap. 1). By this he means that air and blood enter the left and right ventricles of the heart respectively as inspiration occurs and the heart is dilating, and conversely, that venous and arterial blood leave it at the moment of expiration while the heart is contracting. The purpose of both, therefore, is to ensure the movement of blood in the body. A suspicion, however, that Vesalius's views on this point were not entirely Galenic, is unavoidable on the grounds of what happened at the public anatomy which he gave at Bologna in 1540. At his last demonstration, Vesalius vivisected a dog, and after showing the effect of cutting the recurrent nerves, continued:

> Finally, he said, I shall proceed to the heart, so that you shall see its movement, and feel its warmth, thirdly so that you shall here around the ilium feel the pulse with one hand, and with the other the movement of the heart. And please tell me what this movement is, whether the arteries are compressed when the heart is dilated, or whether they in the same time also have the same movement as the heart. . . . Some students asked Vesalius what the true fact about these movements was, what he himself thought, whether the arteries followed the movement of the heart, or whether they had a movement different from that of the heart. Vesalius answered: I do not want to give my opinion, please do feel yourselves with your own hands and trust them.[8]

The first anatomist to call seriously in question the teaching on systole and diastole of the heart was Realdus Columbus in his *De re anatomica*. There when describing the heart, he merely says:

> They call the movement of the heart now diastole, now systole, that is to say, while it dilates and while it constricts.

It is when writing of what can be learned from vivisections, that Columbus records what he himself has seen while watching a heart beat (Bk XIV, p 257):

> In addition to these things which are most beautiful to behold [sc. the movements of the diaphragm], there is another, namely the movement of the heart, how it is enlarged and contracted. If you like, you can also see, in a living anatomy, of what kind is the movement of the arteries, whether indeed it is the same as the movement of the heart, or the opposite. You will find out that while the heart is dilating the arteries are constricted, and again, while the heart is constricting that the arteries are dilated. Of a truth, you will see that when the heart is drawn up and seen to be swollen, then it is constricted. When it decontracts, it falls back as if relaxed, and at that moment the heart is said to be quiescent. This then is the *systole* of the heart, because it undertakes this action more easily and with less labour. But when it transmits [the blood], it needs greater strength. And do not think that this is nonsense, albeit you will find not a few who are convinced in their opinion that the heart is dilated at a time when in fact it is constricted.

That there is something wrong with this passage is evident. The observations on the timing of the arterial pulse are correct, but in the description of the movement of the heart there is a very obvious contradiction: the word *systole*, at the end, is applied to the moment of the heart's relaxation. Jean Riolan noticed this discrepancy and assumed, as a result, that Columbus had no clear idea of the true nature of systole and diastole, and there have been others who have followed Riolan's lead. But that this is not the case is clear from the text itself. It should be remembered that Columbus is looking at the heart of a living dog, lying on its back on the dissecting table. From the angle at which he is looking, he sees the heart swelling and shortening as it constricts. As it relaxes, it falls backwards into the cavity of the chest by the force of gravity. Now these observations are correct and they do contradict the generally accepted theory as he remarks. That he knew full well that *systole* means contraction is evident from the description which he gives elsewhere of the action of the valves of the heart,[9] where it is perfectly clear that he equates constriction with systole, that is, the moment of the expulsion of the blood. This being so, he cannot possibly mean that the heart needs less force in its *systole* and then immediately add that it needs greater force when it transmits the blood, for he knows that this is systole. The error in this passage, therefore, is confined to one word: *systole*. And of this the most obvious and plausible explanation is simply that it is a misprint for *diastole*. The whole of *De re anatomica* is full of misprints, many of which only become apparent on close reading of the text. Their presence is easily explained by the fact that this book was a posthumous publication and it is most unlikely that Columbus saw the proofs of any part of it, with the exception perhaps of Book I. If in this passage we read *diastole* for systole, there is no contradiction in what Columbus says. He is the first anatomist to give a correct description of systole and diastole of the heart. As will be seen,[10] Harvey realised that this was so for he copied the whole of this passage into the notes for his Anatomical Lectures. He noticed that there was something wrong with the text and tried to emend it, but his emendation does not improve the sense. Nevertheless, he was not misled into disbelief of Columbus's real understanding of the heart's movement.

The first anatomist to refer to Columbus's work on systole and diastole was Volcher Coiter, and he was not deceived by the misprint. Like Columbus, Coiter also carried out many experiments on animals and he records his observations on the movement of the heart in his *Externarum et internarum principalium humani corporis partium tabulae atque anatomicae exercitationes observationesque variae*, printed in Nuremberg in 1573. He begins with observations on the movement of the auricles (p. 124):

> For the right understanding of the movement of the heart, living animals are the most suitable, such as nearly all kinds of amphibia, cats, lizards, snakes, and among fish, eels, pike and others of the same kind. I indeed opened the chest of a young living cat. . . . Having cut the pericardium, I saw the double and contrary movement of the heart, that is to say, of the heart [*sc.* the ventricles of the heart] and of its auricles. While the heart was making a beat, the auricles subsided; again, when the heart [*sc.* ventricles] subsided, the auricles were enlarged and filling, so that the diastole of the auricles coincided with the systole of the heart [*sc.* ventricles] and the systole of the auricles with the diastole of the heart [*sc.* ventricles]. The auricles behaved in this manner in diastole: they were seen to be inflated like bladders and when they were fully swollen they acquired a reddish colour, and for a very short space they paused before they hurried into systole; so after their systole they make a short pause before they hasten into diastole. Just as in their diastole the auricles turn red and are swollen because of their repletion with blood

and spirit, so in their systole they grow white and subside, flaccid and shrivelled, and are pulled not a little towards the base of the heart by the force of the heart [*sc.* ventricles].

This far Coiter's observations seem reasonably correct. What is lacking is any reference to the timing of the auricular contractions in relation to those of the ventricles, apart from the general remark that they are alternate. There is no hint of the brief interval after which the ventricular contraction follows the auricular. However, on the whole it seems as though Coiter did distinguish correctly between the systole and diastole of the auricles. It is when he describes the systole and diastole of the ventricles that doubt begins to arise as to whether he really understood what he was watching. It would seem to follow from what he has already said that if he knows that the systole of the auricles coincides with the diastole of the ventricles, and if he is aware of which is the systole of the auricles, then his description of the systole and diastole of the ventricles must be correct. But this is not so. An explanation of his error might lie in a misunderstanding of the timing of the alternate movements of the auricles. Though he is correct in saying that when the auricles are in diastole they are swollen and red, he may not realise that they present this appearance at the end of diastole and also at the beginning of systole. Be that as it may, his description of the movement of the ventricles, though nicely observed, is completely wrong.

> The diastole of the heart [*sc.* of the ventricles] happens in this way: the wrinkled base is constricted and dragged downwards towards the conical tip and what it loses in length it make up for in roundness; the walls of the heart on all sides are distended, the tip is drawn upwards towards the base and it gently strikes against the chest. In this action there is no part or fibre of the heart which is not seen to labour and become wrinkled, for, as the base is dragged downwards and the tip upwards towards the centre of the heart, the ventricles are expanded and the heart is made shorter and rounded. When the diastole is over, it pauses for a moment before it prepares itself for systole, and this is the time which Galen calls the intermediate moment or quiescence between diastole and systole. My first master of pious memory, Regner Praedinius, who was a man of the highest integrity, guileless and of very great erudition and eloquence, was wont to call it διαλεμμα, as if you were to say 'intermission'. After this moment of scarcely comprehensible quiescence, the heart again subsides and becomes thinner, greater in extent, longer, more flaccid and more pale and makes its systole.

In this passage, even if one were to substitute the word 'systole' for 'diastole' and vice-versa, the description would still not be correct. Its muddled nature shows very clearly the difficulty experienced by any anatomist of the time attempting to watch the diverse movements of the heart and their timing and in this way testifies to Harvey's amazing capacity for precise observation. Part of the difficulty for Coiter lies in the fact that he believes that the heart 'attracts' the blood into itself, and consequently, that diastole is not a passive state but an active movement. This is apparent from what he says next with reference to Columbus:

> This behaviour of the heart in diastole and systole would, without any doubt, convert me to the opinion of Realdus Columbus, who thinks that in our diastole blood and spirit are expelled, and that during our systole they are taken in and by no means attracted in (for he holds that blood and spirit slide into the ventricles of the heart while the heart is relaxed), were it not for the fact that the movement of the auricles is the contrary of the movement of the heart [*sc*. ventricles].

Confirmation of this belief that the heart 'attracts' the blood he thought he had found in his observations on the movement of a snake's heart (p. 126):

> In the snake's heart I saw the same things which I have recorded in the heart of a cat and a lizard. The auricles of the heart are dragged inwards with such force in the diastole of the heart that the vena cava which is annexed to the right auricle is also seen to contract. It is abundantly clear from this behaviour that in the heart's diastole, it is with great force that spirit from the pulmonary vein and blood from the vena cava are drawn into the heart.[11]

Coiter now goes on to mention the systole and diastole of the arteries, and because he is wrong about systole and diastole of the heart, he is right when he thinks that their diastole coincides with what he calls the diastole of the heart:

> The arteries are seen at the same time as the heart to make their diastole and systole. . . .

Finally, because of Harvey's observations on the excised heart, it is interesting to notice that Coiter also performed similar experiments:

> Having observed all these things, I cut out the whole heart and after I had for a long time watched its beating with great wonder, I made a long incision into the left ventricle and opened it to learn whether its

pulsation would cease with this sinus or ventricle gashed. But it did not stop pulsating immediately, for the right ventricle persevered a little longer. The same thing happened when I cut the right ventricle. When I opened both ventricles, the mediastinum of the heart and its walls continued to pulsate and particularly the fleshy septum. The last part to pulsate was the base of the heart. This pulsation in the heart of a cat, a snake and a lizard lasted about a quarter of an hour, more or less.

There is no means of knowing for certain whether Harvey had read these observations or not. On the whole, it is unlikely. He quotes Coiter in *De generatione* on the subject of the punctum saliens and makes three references to him in the Anatomical Lectures. One of these references (the abnormal finding of a double urinary bladder in a girl, p. 197), he seems to have taken from the second edition of Bauhin's *Theatrum anatomicum*, for it is an addition to the original text. The two others cannot definitely be traced to Bauhin. Neither has anything to do with the movement of the heart but concerns the number of vertebrae occupied by the gastric region (p. 37), and the number into which the muscles of the back can be divided (p. 377). There is no reference to Coiter in *De motu cordis*. As there are a number of references to Columbus both in the Lectures and in *De motu cordis*, it is reasonable to suppose that if Harvey had used Coiter's work, he would have acknowledged the fact. Though Coiter obviously watched closely the movement of the heart in many different kinds of animals, he unfortunately let preconceived ideas influence his observation; he saw what he expected to see. Though he did observe reptilian hearts, he does not seem to have realised that their behaviour is different from that of the mammalian heart. He did not use the information which could be derived from watching their slow beating to help in the understanding of the exceedingly fast movements of the hearts of cats and dogs. When set beside Coiter's failures in this respect, Harvey's achievements in his observations on mammalian and reptilian hearts are seen in their true perspective. Although Coiter did have some idea about the systole and diastole of the auricles, his observations are incomplete because he failed to realise the advance which could be made by the simple expedient of watching the mammalian heart as it slowed up when nearing the point of death. This Harvey did and set out his findings in *De motu cordis* cap. 2.

During the remainder of the century and indeed up to and beyond the publication of *De motu cordis*, the account given by anatomists of

75

the movement of the heart is traditional and wrong. Not one anatomist as far as I have seen, realised that Columbus was right, that the traditional diastole was in fact systole, that diastole was a passive state and that systole was the essential movement of the heart. Not one, until, Harvey, tested the truth of his observations. Opinion as to whether the systole and diastole of the arteries coincided or not with that of the heart continued likewise to be diverse. To correct Galen on points of anatomical error was one thing; to overturn any part of his doctrine was another. An account of the debate on both these points will be found in the *Historia anatomica* of Laurentius and in its English counterpart, the *Microcosmographia* of Helkiah Crooke, published in London in 1615. There is nothing in either work but much argument based on physiological error. Their reading merely serves to enhance our admiration for Harvey's capacity to cut through this tangle of muddled thinking, abounding in disparate and even contradictory notions, born of imperfect observation and imperfect understanding.

NOTES

1. *Opera*, ed. Kühn. II, pp. 207–08; see also Loeb edition, ed. A. J. Brock, 1916, pp. 321, 323. In the sixteenth-century editions of Galen the reference is to *De nat. fac.*, III, 14; see Galen, *Opera*, Basel 1549, vol. I, col. 1180. A further reference to the ventricular pores occurs in *De usu partium*, VI, 17: Quamobrem quae vena in cor infigitur, maior ea est, quae ab eodem exoritur, tametsi ea fusum iam a cordis calore sanguinem recepit. Sed quoniam multus is per septum medium, et quae in ipso sunt foramina, in sinistrum ventriculum transumitur, factum iure est, ut quae vena in pulmonem inseritur, ea minor esset vena sanguinem in cor introducente (Basel, I, col. 581; Kühn, III, p. 497).

2. An erroneous but commonly held opinion which derived from the post-mortem appearance of the heart; cf. Bauhin, *Theatrum anatomicum*, 1605, II, 21, p. 419. Harvey seems to have disagreed for he omitted this sentence when copying Bauhin's text into his notes, see his *Anatomical Lectures*, p. 256n.

3. The text here reads 'vena cava and pulmonary vein', but that this is an error probably due to the printer is evident from what follows.

4. The text has *arterialis vena* in error for *arteria venalis*.

5. *De medicina veteri et nova*, Basel 1571, p. 91.

6. ed. Willis, p. 19. It would be wrong to think that this is an original piece of Harvey's writing. Much of it, including the reference to Fracastorius is taken, over *verbatim* from the *Historia anatomica* of Laurentius whom Harvey names a little further on.

7. The experiment is twice described by Galen, once in the treatise *An in arteriis natura sanguis contineatur*, and once in his book *On anatomical procedures*, VII, 16 (ed. Singer 1956, pp. 199–200). It is twice referred to by Harvey. Once in the *Anatomical Lectures* (p. 269), where he says that it is impossible to perform, and once, more than thirty years later, in the *Second Disquisition to Riolan* (ed. Willis, pp. 110–11), where he relates how he had performed it and says that 'it supplies nothing in support of the opinion that the coats of the vessel are the cause of the pulse'.

8. *Andreas Vesalius' First Public Anatomy at Bologna, 1540*, ed. Ruben Eriksson, Uppsala and Stockholm, 1959, p. 293.

9. Above, pp. 51-2

10. See below, p. 92.

11. A totally incorrect observation of the movement of the heart.

The Realisation and Publication

Chapter Three

London 1603–1615

HARVEY left Padua some time after April 1602, and it seems likely that early in 1603 he was already settled in London with the intention of practising medicine. In spite of his Paduan diploma, he could not do this without a licence from the College of Physicians. Accordingly, he made a request to be examined and was summoned for the first time by the President and Censors of the College on 4 May 1603. He was the only candidate to be examined on that day. 'His replies to all questions were entirely satisfactory. . . . Nevertheless he was put off until another time, with our tacit permission to practise.' While Harvey was in Padua, there had been no outbreak of plague. He had received permission to practise in London at the beginning of one of the worst epidemics of the century, but we do not know whether he availed himself of the College's permission or not. Nothing in his writings suggests that he had ever seen a major epidemic of plague. We do not know whether he stayed in London or went into the country. All that is certain is that in the spring of 1604 he was again in London.

On 2 April 1604, he appeared a second time before the College of Physicians and his answers to the questions put to him were approved.[1] His third examination went off successfully on 11 May, and his fourth on 7 August, when he was admitted as a Candidate. Finally, on 5 October, he took the oath to the College and became a *Permissus* or Licenciate, and was free to practise medicine within the jurisdiction of the College. In November, he was living in a house in the parish of St Martin, Ludgate, and from there, before the year was out, he was married in the church of St Sepulchre to Elizabeth, the daughter of Dr Lancelot Browne, physician to Elizabeth I and James I. Attempts of his father-in-law to get Harvey the post of physician to the Tower met with no success. In 1607, Harvey was admitted Fellow of the College of Physicians, and was formally appointed physician to St Bartholomew's Hospital on 14 October 1609. His duties in this office were to attend the Hospital at least twice a week throughout the year, to examine the sick brought before him in the hall of the Hospital, and to prescribe for them the necessary medicines. Unlike the three surgeons of the Hospital, he was not expected to visit the patients in the wards. For his services as physician, he received an annual salary of £25, and, until 1627, an allowance of 40s. for his livery. The Hospital's physician usually lived in a house on the site, but it was let when Harvey was appointed and he preferred to stay in his own house rather than accept alternative accommodation. When the house did fall vacant in 1626, Harvey again decided not to move, and the Hospital raised his salary to £33 6s. 8d. a year in lieu of his rent-free house. This salary was paid to him for the last time in 1643, and in February 1644, the House of Commons suggested that another should be appointed in his place, for he had 'withdrawn himself from his charge and is retired to the party in arms against the Parliament.'

From 1609 until 1630, however, Harvey's attendance at the Hospital was regular, and his private practice in the City and at the Court increased. In 1618, he was made one of the physicians to James I and his ties with the royal family grew closer, particularly after the accession of Charles I. We know little about Harvey's private practice.[2] It is possible that all his case-notes were destroyed along with so much else when the Parliamentary troops rifled his lodgings in Whitehall early in the Civil War. All that remains for us to judge him by as a physician are references in his books and a few prescriptions. His skill and wisdom as a gynaecologist and obstetrician are plain from remarks he makes in *De generatione*. His prescriptions show him to have been orthodox and conservative in therapeutics. John Aubrey records having heard him say that after the publication of *De motu cordis*, 'he fell mightily in his Practize and that 'twas beleeved by the vulgar that he was crack-brained'. But Aubrey's final judgement of him as a physician: 'All his profession would allowe him to be an excellent Anatomist, but I never heard of any that admired his therapeutique way', may well be wide of the truth.

Harvey's great love in London was for the College of Physicians and his association with it grew closer as the years passed. After being elected a Fellow, he was frequently present at the meetings of Comitia and took an active part in the business of the College. In 1613, he was elected Censor for the first time, and two years later, on 4 August 1615, he was appointed Lumleian lecturer with the obligation to read a series of lectures on certain prescribed books, and, in the following spring, to perform a full-scale public anatomy in the hall of the College.

The Lumleian lectureship had been founded by Lord Lumley and Dr Richard Caldwell in 1582 to provide lectures for surgeons. Because the practice of this art was then in so poor a state that 'many wise men have rather chosen to commit themselves being grievously diseased into the hands of old doting women (having no skill at all, but a little blind experience) than into the hands of a common surgeon', they decided that 'an excellent Reader' should be procured to 'read openly in the heart of the College of Physicians in London in good order all the whole course of the Art and Science of Surgery'. So the College accepted a gift of £40 a year for the stipend of the lecturer and regulations governing the lectureship were drawn up. The course was envisaged as covering a period of six years. Twice a week throughout the year, excepting only the twelve days of Christmas, Holy Week and the week preceding Whitsun, the lecturer was to give a public lecture lasting one hour and on a prescribed textbook of surgery. In the first year he had to read the *Tabulae chirurgicae* of the Florentine surgeon, Horatio Moro. The first three-quarters of an hour were to be spent in interpreting the text in Latin; the last quarter in summarising in English what had been said, as a concession to the little Latin of the surgeons. Every other week the lecturer was to devote one of his lectures to the explanation and interpretation of Oribasius's *De laqueis* and Galen's *De fasciis*, so that the surgeons might learn everything about fractures and dislocations. In the second, third and fourth years, the lecturer was expected to read the works of Johannes Tagaultius, *De tumoribus*, *De vulneribus* and *De ulceribus*, respectively. In the fifth year, the sixth book of the *Epitome* of Paul of Aegina, 'De chirurgia', from cap. 91 to the end, was to be read, and in the sixth year the *De materia chirurgica* of Jacobus Hollerius and, for the second time, the *Tabulae chirurgicae* of Moro. The lecturer might take a holiday each year for four weeks, provided that it was not during any of the Law Terms while the courts were in session. This proviso was necessary because, in addition to his lectures, the lecturer was required to hold a public anatomy in the winter of each year, and the subjects for these anatomies were the bodies of executed malefactors. The anatomy was to last five consecutive days, 'if the body may last so long', before and after dinner. In the first year, the lecturer was to dissect 'the whole human body, particularly all the interior parts', and the expenses of this anatomy were to be borne by the College. In the second year, he was to dissect not the whole body but the parts 'contained between the head and the groins'. Two bodies (presumably, though not specified, one male and one female) were to be used in this anatomy to show all the inward parts, and the lecturer was to enumerate all the muscles, nerves, veins, arteries, cartilages and bones, both 'inside and outside', and explain their origins, courses and insertions, and the purposes for which they were designed, reminding his audience the while of the dangers which can happen to each part from cuts, wounds, bruises and so forth. In the third year, the five-day anatomy was to be devoted to the dissection of a human head and the lecturer was to explain its parts and discourse on the dangers of wounds there occurring. In the fourth year, he was to dissect for five days as before, an arm and a leg. He was to speak of the muscles, nerves, veins, arteries, cartilages, tendons, ligaments and bones, of their origin, course and insertion, and to explain the dangers of wounds to these parts. In the fifth year, he was to spend five days in the winter demonstrating the skeleton and, at the same time, to show the use of the various instruments employed for the setting of bones and the reduction of dislocations. There are no instructions for an anatomy in the sixth year.

Such were the public duties of the Lumleian lecturer, and in scope they are obviously similar to those of the lecturer in surgery and anatomy in the University of Padua. The Lumleian lecturer himself was always a Fellow of the College of Physicians. The scope of the lectures shows that his knowledge of surgery must have been considerable, but it should not, therefore, be supposed that he either practised surgery himself, or indeed even knew how to practise. It was the Company of the Barber-Surgeons which issued licences to practise surgery in the City of London or within a radius of seven miles. The candidate was required to serve an apprenticeship of seven years with an experienced surgeon, during which time he had to acquire practical knowledge and manual dexterity. The lectures were designed to give the surgeons a more academic understanding of their craft. The theoretical knowledge which the lecturer was expected to impart was of the kind that any physician learnt as part of his medical education at any university. The distinction between the theory and practice of surgery is made clear by Johannes Tagaultius. His writings were well known in the London of the time, for they were put together and translated by Thomas Gale, master of surgery, and published in 1586 under the title, *Booke upon the art of Chirurgerie*. There it is written of surgery:

> The Theorike part doth teach and is a science obteined by demonstration and by knowing the principle of the art. This part a man may have, although he never exercise or practise anie parte of the same, as the learned Physitions and other learned men which dailie readeth the principle of Chirurgerie: But the Practike parte of Chirurgerie, is an arte which doth rightlie and redailie, by the administration of the hand use such things as are invented amongst the mechanical arts, which part no man can be perfect in, except he be brought up and exercised in the same. And doth both continuallie see other expert men worke in the same arte and diligentlie observe such things as he doth see wrought.

The surgeon was basically an expert craftsman, and the extent of his art or craft was the curing of diseases and infirmities by the use of his hands. So, in the same book, the four things required of a good surgeon are summed up as follows:

> First, that he be learned and verie skilfull in the principles of his art; secondly, that he be wel brought up under some cunning man, and wel experienced: thirdly, that he be ingenious and wise, fourthly, that he be of good and honest manners, and of a vertuous life.

The great distinction between the physician and surgeon was that the physician did not use his hands. Every physician, however, had to know enough about surgery to be able to advise his patients when surgical intervention was necessary, and to assess the capacities of the surgeon whom he called upon to perform the operation. When post-mortem investigations were undertaken, as they frequently were in the sixteenth and seventeenth centuries, the physician called upon a surgeon to perform the dissection. To assume, as some have done, that because Harvey shows considerable knowledge of some aspects of surgical procedure, he himself practised any form of surgery is completely to misunderstand the custom of the times. His knowledge of surgery was merely such as might have been expected of any Fellow of the College of Physicians of the day, with the only proviso that, as a practising anatomist he knew more about anatomy from his dissections and his animal experiments than many of his colleagues. The 'little silver instruments of surgerie' which he bequeathed to Doctor Scarbrough

85

may perhaps have been his instruments for venesection; they may equally well have been the instruments he used for his experimental work on animals.

The first Lumleian lecturer to be appointed was Dr Richard Forster. He was bidden to travel in Europe for two years and then to begin his series of lectures 'on the first day of the Easter Term which shall be Anno Domini 1588'. He resigned the lectureship on 20 December 1602. The establishment of this lectureship was heralded with joy, and Hollinshed referred to it in his *Chronicle*, saying:

> now may England reioice for those happie benefactors and singular wel willers to their countrie, who furnish hir so in all respects, that now she may as compare for the knowledge of physicke so by means to come to it, with France, Italie, and Spaine. . . .[3]

The College of Physicians had realised from its very early days that it was important for the young Candidates, as well as for the Licentiates and Fellows, to see full-scale anatomies with a certain regularity. An annual anatomical demonstration was accordingly instituted, and to provide subjects for dissection, the College obtained a royal charter from Queen Elizabeth I in 1565, giving it the right to dissect the bodies of criminals hanged in the City of London, in Middlesex or in any county within a radius of sixteen miles. The College's anatomy was held each year in the winter, and one of the Fellows of the College was selected to give it, the choice being determined by seniority. As has been seen, however, the charges of the full-scale Lumleian anatomy were also to be borne by the College, so that it would appear that, in some years at least, the College was expected to bear the cost of two such anatomies. The expenses involved would therefore have been heavy, the difficulty of obtaining material not inconsiderable. It is not surprising that, in the event, the College's and the Lumleian full-scale anatomy seem to have coalesced. In 1599, it was decided that the College's anatomy should be given in alternate years by a Fellow of the College and by the Lumleian lecturer. Attendance at these anatomies was obligatory and default punished by a fine graduated according to status. The change was consequently welcomed, for it diminished the number of compulsory attendances and allowed members of the College more time to devote 'to the more important and pressing business of the College'. In 1602, it was decided that the annual anatomy should thereafter be held at the end of the Hilary Term and not during the earlier part of the winter. Exactly how this worked out in fact is not abundantly clear from the *Annals* of the College. Fellows were appointed in 1609 and 1610 to hold the College's anatomies in 1610 and 1611 respectively. No one was appointed for 1612, but arrangements were made for 1613 to 1616 inclusive. On 24 November 1615, it was decided that Dr Herring should give the College's anatomy lecture at the end of the Hilary Term, 1616, and the next appointment made by the College was on 28 June 1617, when Dr William Harvey was informed that it was his turn to give this lecture in the spring of 1618.

Following his appointment as Lumleian lecturer on 4 August 1615, Harvey gave his first public anatomy in 1616. On this occasion it lasted for three days, presumably before and after dinner, on 16, 17 and 18 April. Harvey himself dated the manuscript containing the notes for his lectures and no further evidence for the date should be required, were it not for the fact that he also says that he delivered these lectures either at the age of thirty-seven, or during his thirty-seventh year, *aetatis suae 37*. As he was born in 1578, this implies either 1614 or 1615, a manifest impossibility having regard to the date of his appointment as Lumleian lecturer. As he does not say that these are the notes for his Lumleian anatomy, we should examine the possibility that they were first used on an earlier occasion, on the assumption that Harvey made a mistake in the date of the year. But, as has already been said, the College's anatomies in those years were not entrusted to Harvey. Moreover, confirmation that 1616 is indeed the correct date may be had from the Sessions Records for Newgate prison, preserved in the Record Office of the City of London. In that year, on Friday, 12 April, all those accused of felonies were summoned before the justices; two were condemned to be hanged for theft, and on one or other, or both, of these bodies Harvey may well have given his anatomy on the following Tuesday, Wednesday and Thursday. In no other of the neighbouring years do the dates of the gaol-delivery coincide with 16, 17 and 18 April. It follows, therefore, that Havey made no mistake about the year in which he gave these lectures for the first time. He had, in fact, just passed his thirty-eighth birthday when he delivered them, but had doubtless been preparing them for more than two weeks.

These notes for his Lectures on the Whole of Anatomy, the *Prelectiones anatomiae universalis*, were used by Harvey on many subsequent occasions. Additions to their original text, written between the lines, in the margins and on originally blank pages, containing as they do references to autopsies and quotations from new books or from new editions of books appearing after 1616, prove that the manuscript of the notes was in his hands until at least 1626. The latest dateable reference is to an edition of a book by Jean Riolan which appeared in that year. One such addition, written on an originally blank page, is the celebrated brief statement of the circulation of the blood. The handwriting is unlike that of the main bulk of the text, and unlike any of Harvey's other additions. Nothing, in fact, in the whole manuscript seems to have been written at the same time as this and there is no reason to suppose that it was added before the publication of *De motu cordis* rather than afterwards. What date may be given to it will be discussed later when the passage itself is considered.[4] The question which cannot be answered is *why* Harvey should have added it to these notes. For many years this passage has constituted a trap for the unwary. Those who have deciphered it, but not the rest of the text, have erroneously believed that already in 1616 Harvey was in full possession of the knowledge of the circulation of the blood, in spite of what he himself says about the growth of his ideas in *De motu cordis*. Since the text of the *Prelectiones* is now in print, it is possible to know precisely what it contains, and how far Harvey had gone in 1616 towards his hypothesis that the blood circulated throughout the whole body. That he had then no idea that this would be his conclusion is obvious.

NOTES

1. On this occasion one of the four examined with Harvey was Thomas Hearne whose doctoral diploma at Padua Harvey witnessed as Councillor on 19 March 1602; see above p. 39, *n*. 19.
2. For details of Harvey's practice of medicine, see Keynes, *Life*, caps 5, 11, 15, 18, etc.
3. Vol. IV, London 1808, p. 498. The reference to Spain is unexpected. Valverde explained in the preface to his textbook which he wrote in Spanish for the express benefit of the physicians and surgeons of his country, that he had used Vesalius's pictures because he did not want to confuse those who read it by including a different and, most likely, indifferent set, for they had no means of verifying what was depicted by comparing it with actual cadavers, dissections being rarely performed in Spain.
4. See below, p. 169.

Chapter Four

The Lectures on the Whole of Anatomy
1616

As the basis for his notes on anatomy, Harvey used the textbook of Caspar Bauhin, the *Theatrum anatomicum*, in its first edition printed at Frankfurt in 1605. The choice was an excellent one. Bauhin's book was the culmination of all his anatomical writings, which he had begun in 1588, and it immediately acquired the well-deserved reputation of being the best textbook available. It contained a systematic account of the subject and referred adequately to all the ancient authorities, Aristotle, Hippocrates, Galen, Avicenna and the rest. It did not ignore the moderns or their more recent discoveries. Provided these discoveries were sufficiently authenticated by reference to observation and experiment, they were included in the text (a case in point is the discovery by Fabricius of the valves of the veins); if not, they were relegated to a reference in a footnote. The book did not go into too much detail over anatomical controversy and did not waste time in argument and debate on abstruse and unprovable opinions. It mentioned anatomical abnormalities and pathological findings. It was born of Bauhin's many years of experience of teaching anatomy in the University of Basel. Its footnotes betray the scholarly mind of its author and constitute, by their references, a very encyclopaedia of the anatomical knowledge of the day. Bauhin himself made no great anatomical discoveries. Though he believed that he was the first to describe the ileo-caecal valve, for long called after him *valvula Bauhini*, this was probably not the case. His great contribution to anatomy was the reform which he introduced into the nomenclature, particularly into that of muscles. As he explains, because it is very easy to make mistakes in the enumeration of muscles,

89

if they are merely called first, second, third, and so forth, and because different anatomists term different muscles in this way and do not agree in the order of the enumeration, Bauhin decided that it was better to use another kind of terminology. So he named some muscles according to their substance (semimembranosus, etc.), others according to their shape (deltoid, scalene, etc.), some according to their origin (arytenoideus etc.), others according to their origin and insertion (styloglossus, crycothyroideus, etc.). Some he named according to the number of their heads (biceps, triceps), some according to their amount (vastus, gracilis), some according to their position (pectoralis, etc.) and others according to their use (supinator, pronator, etc.). The advantages of this system over the old method were so obvious that it was adopted by all subsequent anatomists. At the time when Harvey used his book, Bauhin was still professor at Basel. Like Harvey he had in his youth been for a while a student at Padua and a pupil of Fabricius. He died at Basel 5 December 1624. He was, as Harvey called him, 'a rare industrious man' and a firm believer in the precept that truth demonstrable to the beholder outweighs the opinions of the authorities.

Bauhin's book was primarily designed for students and not for professors of anatomy, and as such it was obviously suitable for Harvey's use for his own lectures. For the basic description of the parts of the body on which he had to comment as they were dissected, Harvey therefore used Bauhin's text, even on occasions copying it verbatim into his notes. At other times he wrote only a few essential words which are meaningless unless their context is known. Harvey's own remarks and opinions, interspersed among the quoted material, are frequently, but not always, prefixed by the initials WH. His disagreements he usually marks by the simple sign X. To read the text of the *Prelectiones*, therefore, and assert that such and such was Harvey's opinion is only to be undertaken advisedly. Instead of Harvey's views in any particular sentence, it is possible that Bauhin's views are being rehearsed, and that Harvey is not in agreement with the statement he has just written down may only be revealed a little further on in the text. As a result, in one or two places, actual contradictions will be found, because Harvey was contradicting not himself, but the views of Bauhin's textbook.[1] Harvey's views have to be disentangled from non-original material. Moreover, it must not be forgotten that Harvey's notes were intended to serve as a basis for a spoken commentary and do not necessarily represent everything that he said. They are not a finished piece of writing and only from time to time are there passages of continuous prose. These passages are usually those in which Harvey is giving an account of his own views and discussing a particular point. The references which Harvey gives to other authorities, though frequently to be found in Bauhin's footnotes, are not always so derived. This is particularly so in the case of his references to Aristotle. That Harvey used in this way another's book for his own lectures should cause no surprise, for it is in the tradition of all the medical teaching of the period. His lectures were intended to teach the basic essentials of the subject. There was not time to discuss every new opinion, for the whole of the anatomy of the human body had to be described and demonstrated in the compass of three days.

Harvey's views on the movement of the heart and blood have to be collected from different parts of the lectures, from his remarks on veins and arteries, from his description of the brain, but chiefly from what he has to say concerning the heart and lungs. His description of the heart follows the traditional pattern and is for the most part directly derived from Bauhin. In some places the description is little more than perfunctory. He pauses to insert some of his opinions and some experimental or pathological findings, but nothing relevant to his views on the heart's movement.

It is with what he has to say on this subject, a little further on in the notes, that he begins to reveal the state of his ideas in 1616. In a brief statement he summarises the accepted teaching:

> The movement of the heart: it is commonly believed that when the point of the heart is pulled up towards the base and the ventricles are dilated, that this is diastole, and on the contrary that when the heart is again stretched out that this is systole. Therefore, it is thought that the heart strikes the chest in diastole and that in diastole when the heart is dilated the artery is also dilated. It is also believed that the chief movement of the heart is diastole and that death befalls in systole and that from diastole comes the inner quiescence of the heart and pulse (p. 265).

The passage is merely a summing up of Bauhin's statements. Harvey then continues:

> I have observed these things for hours together and I have not been able easily to distinguish between them either by sight or by touch. Wherefore I would now lay them before you that you may see them with your own eyes and judge for yourselves. It seems to me rather that either

91

what they call diastole is the contraction of the heart, and consequently has been ill defined, or else X it is what they say it is; or at least in diastole the fleshy wall of the heart is thickened while the ventricles are in truth compressed.

The 'X' here certainly implies 'with this I do not agree'. At this point Harvey copied out from Columbus's book, *De re anatomica*, his description of systole and diastole of the arteries and of the heart, including the misprint and making an alteration and a mistake:

Columbus, p. 474, says that while the heart is dilating the arteries are constricted, and again, while the heart is constricting that the *veins* are dilated. NB that when the heart is drawn up and seen to be swollen, then it is constricted. When it decontracts, it falls back as if relaxed and at that moment the heart is said to be quiescent and *it is said that* this is the systole of the heart because it undertakes this action more easily and with less labour, but when it sends out the blood it needs much greater strength. And do not think that this is nonsense, albeit you will find not a few who are convinced in their opinion that the heart is dilated at a time when in fact it is constricted.

First, the mistake. Harvey has written *veins* for arteries. Columbus's text has neither word at the end of this sentence as none is necessary; arteries is clearly inferred from the first half. But, after the full stop, the next word, printed very close, is *Verū*. This I suggest Harvey simply misread in a moment of careless copying.[2] As for the misprint and the alteration, they are linked. Seeing that 'systole' in the context makes nonsense of Columbus's statement, Harvey has tried to get over the difficulty by relating it to the commonly accepted view which Columbus is contradicting. His alteration does not improve the meaning of the passage, but nevertheless Harvey realised what Columbus was really saying. His acknowledgements to Columbus in *De motu cordis* put the matter beyond doubt. That by 1616 Harvey was in a position to know that Columbus's view was the correct one, is evident from what follows.

After quoting Columbus, Harvey again remarks on the difficulty of observing correctly:

See how hard and difficult it is to distinguish either by sight or by touch between dilatation and contraction and to say of what nature is systole and what diastole.

To obviate some of the difficulties occasioned by the rapidity of the heart's movement, Harvey observed it in cold-blooded creatures, and of its action in fish he is quite certain:

> In fish it is evident that the heart is made smaller during the movement of lifting itself up and the blood is thrust forth (p. 267).

As this observation confirms his suspicions, he now takes the bold step of setting up as an hypothesis the statement that systole is the essential movement of the heart, thus contradicting contemporary opinion and following Columbus. For the purpose of his argument he chooses the very action that was thought to be characteristic of diastole, the apex beat of the heart, and equates this with the moment of systole. From this certain observations follow:

> The action of lifting itself up is the proper movement of the heart for it is first made active and then is relaxed and wanting in vigour. If the action of lifting itself up be said to be systole, then 1. the heart strikes the chest in the action of lifting itself up; 2. from soft it indeed becomes hard, so that it can be felt only when it is lifting itself up; the vein appears larger; 3. the auricles are seen to contract themselves and become white in colour, and the blood is thrust forth . . . (pp. 265-7).

Coiter had also remarked that the auricles become white and subside when they go into systole. It seems as though Harvey is here omitting the very brief time interval between the auricular and ventricular contractions. When he says that the vein appears larger, he presumably means that the vena cava swells as the entry of its blood into the heart is momentarily halted. No one but Harvey seems to have mentioned the fact that the ventricles are hard to the touch as they pass into systole. Their whiteness evidently fixed his attention for he refers to their colour again later:

> the heart is whiter and more glistening in the action of lifting itself up, as can be seen in frogs, fish, etc. (p. 269).

To test the validity of the hypothesis which the observations seem to support there follows the simple experiment of making an incision into a ventricle:

> If the heart has been pierced, the blood flows out, spurts out, as the heart lifts itself up, and therefore this is systole, and at the same time the pulse of the artery can be perceived (p. 267).

93

In passing it is interesting to notice that Harvey is here using the method of advancing knowledge originally advocated by Aristotle. It was subsequently developed by the Aristotelian philosophers of Padua and is sometimes described by the cant phrase 'up and down the ladder'. Certain observations suggest an hypothesis. The validity of the hypothesis is then tested by precise observation and experiment. Its truth is thus demonstrated. This is what Harvey means when he says in setting out his conclusions that he has proceeded 'according to the strictest form'.

> This error has been current for a very long time and therefore I have proceeded according to the strictest form because the subject is so ancient a one and has been studied by so many great men. First, what they call diastole, be it systole or diastole, is the thickening of the fleshy mass of the heart only, and the contraction of the ventricles. Second, the lifting up of the heart, again whether you call it systole or diastole, is the proper movement of the heart as opposed to its relaxation. Third, at the moment of rising up, the blood spurts out and the pulse occurs . . .; as in a glove. . . . At the time of relaxation the blood enters the ventricles and therefore they are filled with blood of a more vivid colour.

From the outset, Harvey seems to be thinking of the movement of the heart in the terms of the movement of muscle. This was also a subject in which Fabricius had taken particular interest. Although Harvey was later (in the notes which he wrote in 1627 for his projected treatise on animal movement) to disagree with Fabricius over what was the contractile element in muscle, they both held that contraction was its essential movement. Harvey, moreover, thought that contraction was due to the fleshy fibre of muscle. Consequently, Harvey says here of the heart that it 'is made of a fibrous substance for the purpose of contracting and for this it needs strength'. He analyses its movement in the terms of its structure of longitudinal and transverse fibres and reaches a conclusion different from that of Vesalius, to whom he does not here refer:

> when the fibres of the heart are contracted lengthways the walls of the heart are thickened, when the fibres are contracted widthways, the walls are compressed, as happens in the muscles of the abdomen (p. 271).

As he does not make the point in the notes, we cannot be completely certain whether at this date he had already jettisoned the erroneous notion that the explanation of the heart's action lay in the contraction and relaxation of the longitudinal and transverse fibres alternately. In *De motu cordis* it is plain that he had done so:

> Neither is it to be allowed ... that the heart is moved only by its straight fibres, and so whilst the top is brought near to the bottom, the sides of it are dilated round about and do acquire the form of a little gourd and so take in the blood, for, along all the lines of all the fibres that it has, the heart is at one and the same time stiffened and gathered together, and the outside and the substance of it are thickened and dilated, rather than the ventricles; and while the fibres running from the top to the bottom do draw the top towards the base, the sides of the heart do not incline to an orbicular figure, but rather the contrary, just as every fibre circularly placed does in its contraction tend to become straight; so, like the fibres of all the muscles, whilst they [*sc.* the longitudinal fibres of the heart] are contracted and shortened in length so are they extended in breadth and are thickened after the same fashion as the bellies of the muscles (p. 22, altered).

Between 1616 and 1628, Harvey had spent much time on the study of the behaviour of muscles, and the knowledge of how they act informs his description of the heart's action.

In *De motu cordis*, Harvey separates the problem of the movement of the arteries from that of the heart. In the Lectures the problems are not dissociated in this logical manner. Several times he repeats the observation that the pulsation of the artery is synchronous with the systole of the heart, as can be seen in the quotations already given. He has, moreover, proved it experimentally by cutting arteries. He therefore concludes that the pulse is caused by the systole of the heart:

> Hence the arterial pulse does not come from some innate pulsative faculty, but from the thrusting forth of the blood by the heart (p. 269). So the heart while it is pulsating is driving on the blood, and the pulse is the driving on of the blood, and also a certain driving in of the blood, as in a glove (p. 271).
> Action of the heart: thus relaxed receives blood; contracted, scups it over. The whole of the body responds to the artery as my breath in a glove (p. 273).

So the arteries do not expand like bellows and draw the blood into them as bellows draw air, but are forcibly expanded like bladders by the impetus of the blood driven into them from the heart. What is lacking here, by comparison with *De motu cordis*, is the statement that the pulse of the arteries reflects the rhythm and volume of the heart's contractions. Also lacking are the observations relating to the cessation of the arterial pulse when the ventricles cease to contract, and to the possibility of interfering with it by compression. Nor does he yet make use of his observations on aneurysms, though when discussing the reason for the pulsation of the venous sinuses of the brain, he glances at a cognate problem:

> the pulse is made by the arteries and the spirits, and because of this the whole brain seems to pulsate because it is like a quagmire. Just as suppuration cannot be arrested in the case of an imposthume, if it be near an artery, so it is with the pulsation of the arteries (p. 309).

By 1616, Harvey knew everything that was essential about the movement of the auricles, but his remarks are based on observation rather than experiment.

> The pulse begins from the auricles and progresses to the tip of the heart . . . (p. 267).
> . . . the ventricles of the heart answer to the movement of the auricles, so that the heart itself [sc. the ventricles] drives out the blood which has just been driven into it (p. 269).

He does not mention the experiment of cutting off the point of the heart to watch the blood escaping at each auricular contraction as described in De motu cordis, cap. 4. He seems to have done some, but not all, the work on the dying heart, but he has observed the increasing slowness with which the ventricular contraction follows the auricular in a heart in this condition:

> The auricle arouses the sleepy heart. The heart in process of answering responds at first well enough, then quite evidently after a little delay, but finally not at all (p. 267).

What is lacking here is any reference to the occurrence of two or three auricular beats before the answering ventricular contraction in a heart on the point of death. But while watching the dying heart, he has seen that as it contracts it twists to the left, a movement which no anatomist before him seems to have noticed:

> When the heart replies tardily to the movement of the auricle, it twists its point a little towards the left (p. 267).

Also from his work on the dying heart, he knows that the right auricle is the last part to pulsate (p. 257), and he has performed the experiment on a dead pigeon:

> A whole hour after a pigeon was dead, its right auricle was pulsating under my finger (p. 267).

This experiment is described in detail in *De motu cordis*, cap. 4. He has made some observations on the hearts of slow-blooded creatures and describes the heart of a fish as having 'as it were a pool of blood' (p. 251). Lastly, he has seen the ventricles continue to pulsate after a heart has been excised, and he has also noticed that even isolated strips of the tissue of the heart retain for a while their movement:

> . . . the heart pulsates after the auricles have been cut off. . . . Even in strips cut from the heart, dilatation is seen to occur, in accordance with the behaviour of flesh [*sc.* fleshy muscle], and so it is unavoidable that the ventricles should be constricted (p. 267).

By contrast with this, Coiter's observations on the excised heart are meaningless.

We may conclude, therefore, that by 1616 Harvey's observations on the movement of the heart were well advanced, and included a study of the behaviour of the auricles and of the ventricles. The observations had been collected from vivisections of slow-blooded creatures, frogs and fish, from birds and probably from the usual experimental animals, dogs and cats. In particular he had made much use of the dying heart, for it had the obvious advantage of allowing him to watch its movements as it were in slow motion. It is strange that no anatomist before him seems to have exploited this simple means of overcoming the difficulty arising out of the speed of the beating of mammalian heart. A certain number of these observations Harvey had tested experimentally, and he had reached the conclusion that systole and diastole were the reverse of what was generally believed, that the arterial pulse was due to the impulse of blood driven into the arteries by the contraction of the heart and, consequently, that the diastole of the arteries coincided with the systole of the heart. But as yet these ideas had not been marshalled in any coherent or logical form, as they were to be in *De motu cordis*. There is, therefore, no summary of them in the Lectures as there is in the fifth chapter of the book. Here Harvey uses again only two points which he had made in the Lectures: the first is the observation, already quoted, that as the heart contracts it turns a little to the left; the other concerns the interventricular septum and will be discussed later.

At this stage it becomes clear that Harvey's analysis of the heart's movement has led him to the acceptance of the truth of Columbus's hypothesis that the blood from the right ventricle passes to the left by way of the pulmonary artery, the lungs and the pulmonary vein.

> From these things it is evident WH that the action of the heart in so far as it is an instrument of movement, is to send the blood from the vena cava into the lungs through the pulmonary artery, and from the lungs through the pulmonary vein into the aorta. When the heart is relaxed, which happens first, there is an entering into it of blood into the right ventricle from the vena cava, and into the left from the pulmonary vein. When it is lifted up, or contracted, it drives out the blood as it were by force from the right ventricle into the lungs and from the left ventricle into the aorta, and this is the reason for the arterial pulse (p. 271).

It will be noticed that Harvey takes the presence of blood in the pulmonary vein as an accepted fact. It is, I think, a little surprising that this is all that Harvey has to say on the pulmonary transit of the blood. As has been seen, he did not learn of it from Fabricius in Padua; it was by no means generally accepted as true by 1616. Presumably he was convinced by the evidence of the competence of the valves of the heart that Columbus was right, yet, as will be seen, this is not a point on which we can be certain, in view of what he says in these Lectures of the pulmonary vein. However, he does accept it and for some reason sees no cause to discuss it further. He makes no reference to fuliginous vapours, almost as if they were beneath contempt, and his account is uncluttered with any notions of vital spirits and speculations on the place of their generation. It is the practical anatomist who is speaking.

All that can be said of Harvey's position in 1616, then, is that he is in the forefront of contemporary physiological thought. He has tested the latest theories and is convinced of their truth, but he has not yet gone beyond this. Nor do I think that he was then aware that various other pieces of knowledge of which he was in possession were clues to the solution of the puzzle. If we consider the use that he makes in *De motu cordis*, cap. 6, of his observations on the movement of the blood in animals having hearts with only one ventricle and no lungs, and also in the foetal heart, it would seem that in 1616 he was not aware of the significance he would later attach to his work on both these kinds of hearts. As his observations on them in the Lectures are, at the best, random, we do not know the extent of his work on them by this date. The observations on the heart of fish found in the Lectures and repeated in this chapter of *De motu cordis* concern the pool of blood which is analogous to an auricle, that is, the sinus venosus (p. 251), and the statement that the pulse is not found in fish except in the pipe or vessel analogous to an artery, that is the ventral aorta (p. 255). We can have no clear idea of his work on the foetal heart at this date because, after the barest description of the vessels, derived directly from Bauhin's textbook, he dismisses the whole subject saying: 'But of these things and of their uses I will speak more exactly when I discuss the foetus' (p. 263). The notes for this discussion are not known to be extant. He describes the auricles in the foetus as being 'pools of blood' (p. 263), and he cites one observation which he used later in *De generatione* (Ex. LI, p. 279):

> I have seen . . . a heart exceedingly white, its auricles purple and filled with blood (p. 127).

There is only one remark on the foramen ovale and the ductus arteriosus which will also be found in *De motu cordis*, cap. 6, and it is to the effect that these passages often remain open after weaning and in some animals which are not perfect (an Aristotelian notion not to be confused with our modern sense), they are even always so (p. 263).

Moreover, Harvey's account of the movement of the heart in the Lectures is not quite as free of all Galenic notions as the foregoing summary implies. In spite of everything he says about the heart impelling the blood by its systolic contraction and his consequent apparent belief in diastole as a passive state, he has not as yet entirely jettisoned the idea of the attractive power of the heart. It would seem that the movement of the vena cava, jolted by the contraction of the heart, had been observed, and that it is to this that Coiter alludes when he speaks of this vein as being 'seen to contract'.[3] But as this moment was mistakenly believed to coincide with the heart's filling, it was thought that the movement of the vena cava denoted the force of the attractive power of the heart by which the blood was sucked into the ventricles. To this belief Harvey alludes twice in the Lectures. When he is enumerating the things which follow from the hypothesis that the rising up of the heart is the moment of its systole (p. 109), his fourth point, omitted above, is:

at the same moment that the arterial pulse can be felt by touch, the vena cava is as it were attracted, *quasi attrahitur vena cava.* [4]

If we translate *attrahitur* as 'attracted', one of its possible meanings, then it seems as though this is a direct reference to the traditional theory. If, on the other hand, we translate it as 'dragged down', an equally possible meaning, then this is simply the observation of a physiological fact. And here there is no evidence available to resolve the dilemma. The second reference is equally ambiguous. It also occurs in connection with remarks on the arterial pulse, and it is linked with the only allusion that Harvey makes throughout the Lectures to the valves in the veins. He has been reflecting on the fact that the arteries have to be of sufficient strength to withstand the impetus of the blood as it is driven into them, and he continues:

> Hence also, neither the vena cava nor the pulmonary vein is of such a structure because they do not pulsate, but rather they may be said to suffer an attraction [*sed potius attrahi*, or 'to be dragged down'], and this because the valves set in a contrary direction break off the pulse both in the heart and in the other veins (p. 273).

Coupled with the fact that Harvey is here about to attribute to the valves a use which is both traditional and false, it may be that he is indeed thinking in terms of the force of attraction felt by the vena cava. In the next sentence he says:

> WH and for this reason, the veins have very many valves opposed to the heart, while the arteries have none except in the exit from the heart in contrary fashion. Hence these veins are capable of pulsating and these indeed are not (p. 273).

The valves in the veins had been described in detail by Bauhin; indeed, as has been said, he was one of the first to incorporate their description into a textbook for students. And Harvey himself had probably seen Fabricius's demonstration of them while he was in Padua. Yet in the Lectures they are nowhere described, neither in the *Prelectiones* nor in their sequel, *De musculis*, where they could easily have been included in the section on the veins of the leg. Their use is only this once summarily stated and neither questioned nor even discussed. If Harvey thinks that their use is to break off the pulse in the veins, as the valves of the heart break off the pulse, then it follows by implication that he thinks that their use is to delay the flow of blood in the veins and this is what Fabricius had believed. It is a belief totally inconsistent with the hypothesis that the blood circulates throughout the whole body. He is thinking of venous blood as leaving the heart, not returning to the heart. If, therefore, Harvey had not yet changed his opinion as to their use, it is unlikely that he had already formulated any hypothesis concerning the general circulation of the blood. From the negative evidence of the Lectures, it would seem that he had not even begun to realise the importance of these valves or to question their use. That this is a crucial point in the development of Harvey's ideas is plain from the fact that Robert Boyle says, on two occasions, that Harvey told him, 'in the only Discourse I had with him', that it was the consideration of the valves in the veins that first 'hinted' to him, or 'induced him to think of', the circulation of the blood. 'When he took notice that the Valves in the Veins of so many several parts of the Body, were so Plac'd that they gave free passage to the Blood Towards the Heart, but oppos'd the passage of the Venal Blood the contrary way: he was invited to imagine that so Provident a Cause as Nature had not so Plac'd so many valves without Design: and no Design seem'd more probable, than That, since the Blood could not well, because of the interposing Valves, be Sent by the Veins to the Limbs, it should be sent through the Arteries, and return through the veins, whose valves did not oppose its course that way.'[5] In 1616, Harvey's consideration of the valves of the veins had not begun.

What Harvey has to say about the interventricular septum in the Lectures shows that he was, at best, divided in his mind.

> Some think that the blood passes across through the septum of the heart, the dividing wall ,which is gibbous from the right side and concave from the left, and therefore they say that the septum is porous which X. Bauhin, however, says that the vents were conspicuous in the heart of an ox which had been boiled (p. 261).

It was this heart of an ox, it will be remembered, that had made Bauhin change his mind about the pulmonary transit of the blood. Harvey certainly contradicts the statement that the septum is porous, for this is the meaning of his X, but he seems to have been troubled by Bauhin's finding. It was, after all, possible at this date to hold the opinion that although most of the blood went through the lungs to the left ventricle, nevertheless a little seeped through the invisible pores. Only Columbus denied it utterly.

Although Columbus discovered the pulmonary transit of the blood, there is no reason to suppose that he queried the notion of blood ebbing and flowing in the other parts of the body, or the belief that the veins carried natural blood from the liver to the parts for their nourishment. His observations on the pulmonary vein and his experiments proved that it contained blood and not air, and his recognition of the competence of the valves of the heart led him to reject the notion of the two-way movement of the blood in this vein. But this did not lead him to question the validity of the notion of the two-way movement of blood and chyle in the branches of the portal vein. Some anatomists who partially accepted Columbus's theory but did not understand its essential feature, the competence of the valves of the heart, kept the place of the generation of the vital spirits in the heart and consequently allowed a two-way passage of blood through the pulmonary vein: of natural blood inwards to be made vital, and of vital blood outwards for the use of the lungs. The suspicion that Harvey himself in 1616 was in this category is roused by his remark on the pulmonary vein: 'Both on account of its office and its origin it may be likened to the portal vein' (p. 261). True, this statement is copied from Bauhin, but Harvey does not contradict it either by his usual X or by a comment, and we are at a loss to know what he really thought.

If we turn to what he has to say on the portal vein, it is obvious that he still held the Galenic notion concerning its use, and consequently accepted the idea of a two-way motion through it. Speaking of the omentum he says: 'it bears the veins from the portal vein to the stomach and the spleen' (p. 79), and of the stomach: 'it receives veins from the splenic branch of the portal vein and they bring in blood and take off chyle' (p. 81). His discussion of concoction in the liver and in the spleen also illustrates the fact that he is still thinking in Galenic terms. Having given the various opinions about the spleen, which was a major subject of controversy at the time, and having rejected them, Harvey gives his own views:

> Because animals like man eat food made up of different parts of which some are of easy concoction and others of more difficult, some of good juice and others of a juice which is black, cold and dry, for the former the liver is necessary; but that part which runs back to the portal veins (where the separation of the bile also occurs) is diverted and attracted to the spleen where it can be received, concocted and perfected by means of the abundant heat and loose texture of the part. And this is seen to

be proved by the structure of the veins, for if the spleen receives the juice through this splenic branch and from the portal vein of the liver, then the spleen is thus situated as if it were a pendant from the liver to receive from it and to be subservient to it (p. 129).

This description should be compared with what Harvey has to say on the subject in *De motu cordis*, cap. 16.[6]

To continue to enumerate the passages in the Lectures in which Harvey makes statements inconsistent with the hypothesis that the blood circulates throughout the body would be tedious and unilluminating. In general terms, his position in 1616 is clear. His experimental work and his observations have led him to confirm Columbus's views on systole and diastole of the heart. He is quite clear about the manner of its action and the fact that it drives the blood into the arteries, so that diastole of the arteries coincides with the systole of the heart. His views on the pulmonary transit of the blood are not explained but he seems to accept it. He gives no indication of understanding the competence of the valves of the heart and he has not begun to think about the significance of the valves in the veins. He had not yet gone beyond the work of Columbus. A mass of data is, however, accumulating, but it is unorganised and its significance is not yet understood.

NOTES

1. Dr J. S. Wilkie in his review of my edition of the *Prelectiones* has made this mistake; *History of Science*, 4 (1965), pp. 119–20.
2. As I did myself in a moment of careless reading. These remarks relate, of course, to the edition printed at Frankfurt in 1593, the edition used by Harvey.
3. See above, p. 74.
4. My translation of this sentence in *The Anatomical Lectures*, p. 267, is wrong as I had not then understood its significance.
5. *A Disquisition about the Final Causes of Things*, London 1688, p. 157.
6. See below pp. 145–6, *n.* 14

Chapter Five

The Discovery 1619–1625

IN the letter addressed to Dr Argent and which serves as a Preface to *De motu cordis*, Harvey wrote, in words which are now famous:

> I did open many times before, worthy Mr Doctor, my opinion concerning the motion and use of the heart and Circulation of the blood new in my lectures; but being confirm'd by ocular demonstration for nine years and more in your sight, evidenced by reasons and arguments, freed from the objections of the most learned and skilfull Anatomists, desired by some, and most earnestly required by others, we have at last set it out to open view in this little Book . . . (p. ix).

For the previous fifty years and more, it had been common practice for anatomists to introduce their books in this manner to the public. They do not wish to appear arrogant or to seek comparison with the great names of the past; they are diffident about the value of their own work, and so they explain that in allowing publication they have yielded to the express wish of some friend or to the importunate demands of their students. But because Harvey's letter is thus conventional, there is no need to doubt its sincerity or the truth of what it says. Dr John Argent, then President of the College of Physicians, was Harvey's 'very dear friend' of many years' standing. He had been present at Harvey's first examination by the College in 1603 and they had served the College's affairs together on many occasions. The President of the College of Physicians would out of courtesy have been one of the first to be informed of Harvey's discoveries; out of courtesy the book would have been dedicated to him. When the President and the friend were united in one person, the probability that he knew every detail of the discovery is increased. From references to him in the *Prelectiones*, it is quite clear that they exchanged views:

> I have seen, as Dr Argent will bear witness, a body with all parts perfected yet with a liver unformed; a heart fashioned with auricles but the liver ill-made and a shapeless mass; a heart exceedingly white, its auricles purple and filled with blood (p. 127).

So Dr Argent saw some of Harvey's dissections of the foetus and he communicated to Harvey some of his pathological findings:

> Yet in hydrocephalus Dr Argent reports that he found the whole brain consumed and nothing left but the meninges (p. 319);

or his experiences in practice:

> See also Dr Argent who said that a stone ate out his passage in the flank (p. 173).

When, therefore, Harvey says that he has been demonstrating the circulation of the blood for 'nine years and more', these words are to be taken literally as a statement of the truth. There is no conceivable reason why Harvey should be inventing.[1]

The date of Harvey's discovery is then attached by him to some time about 1619. But this does not necessarily mean any more than that he then began to think that the evidence which he had accumulated seemed to point towards the hypothesis that the blood circulated throughout the whole of the body. After that would come experiments designed to test its truth, argument and discussion, objections refuted by more experiments, the understanding of the relevance of more observations perhaps already made, so that slowly by observation, vivisection, demonstration and argument, the truth of the whole became plain. The process was not accomplished in the twinkling of an eye. When it was complete we do not know. In *De motu cordis*, Harvey says 'some years before', some years that is before 1628, and perhaps we might hazard a cautious guess that 1625 is approximately the right date. Then Harvey had had to persuade the College of Physicians of the truth of his views, or at least to withhold their active censure. In the seventeenth century, the College of Physicians was the custodian of the truth of medical knowledge, and therefore of Galen's teaching, responsible for the training of new physicians and ever-watchful lest error should be disseminated. It still fined its members for teaching contrary to Galen.

Harvey was a Fellow and his discovery was not some trifling rectification of an anatomical error made by Galen; his discovery showed that the fundamental basis of Galenic doctrine was at fault. In the event it was to bring down the whole edifice of Galenic medicine, so carefully guarded over the centuries, and this Harvey perceived. His caution and his hesitancy are not difficult to understand.

> And since this Book alone does affirm the blood to pass forth and return through unwonted tracts, contrary to the received way through so many ages of years insisted upon and evidenced by innumerable, and those the most famous and learned men, I was greatly afraid to suffer this little Book, otherwise perfect some years ago, either to come abroad, or go beyond the Sea, lest it might seem an action too full of arrogancy, if I had not first propounded it to you, confirm'd it by ocular testimony, answer'd your doubts and objections, and gotten the President's verdict in my favour; yet I was perswaded if I could maintain what I proposed in the presence of you and our College, having been famous by so many and so great men, I needed so much the lesse to be afraid of others, and that only comfort, which for the love of truth you did grant me, might likewise be hoped for from all who were Philosophers of the same nature (pp. x–xi).

Then there was the problem of publication. In the seventeenth century, new findings and new ideas were frequently discussed in letters exchanged between learned men, for there was no equivalent of our modern scientific periodicals. Fabricius, it will be remembered, had allowed his 'monographs' to accumulate and had waited years before publication in order to avoid error. Harvey's step was, therefore, a bold one and it is not surprising that he took what precautions he could to ensure for his book a fair-minded judgement. If all his colleagues in the College did not support his views, at least some did and the others seem to have refrained from public criticism.

It is strange and sad that although the members of the College of Physicians must have seen Harvey's demonstrations, not one is known to have left any record concerning them. Yet some even assisted him:

> I can call most of you, being worthy of credit, as witnesses of those observations from which I gather truth, or confute error, who saw many of my Dissections, and in the ocular demonstrations of these things which I here assert to the senses, were us'd to stand by and assist me (p. x).

Unless in the course of time, more documents are discovered, letters or papers of these members of the College, the problem as to the precise date of Harvey's discovery will remain insoluble.

Harvey's statements which seem to point to the years between 1619 and perhaps 1625 as being crucial to the discovery make the notes for the Lectures on the Whole of Anatomy even more incomprehensible. There is, as has been said, evidence to show that he added to them over a period of ten years, up to and including 1626, that is during the very years of his discovery. Yet these additions give no clue. Not one would lead us to suppose that he was in possession of the facts of the circulation. Strangest of all is the addition made in 1626. The addition of Riolan's *Anthropographiae*, printed in that year, contains a description which does not appear in the earlier edition, of how when he blew into the spermatic, that is the ovarian, veins of a woman, he saw that the arteries along the uterus were inflated together with the veins. This description Harvey copied out and added the comment, *An contra?* 'Or does the reverse occur?' In his *De generatione* of 1651, Harvey refers again to this same passage and contradicts it, saying that this 'is a prevalent argument for the Circulation of the Blood which was my invention; for it clearly doth evince a passage from the Arteries into the Veins, but no retreat from the Veins into the Arteries again.' By 1626 one might have expected to find Harvey contradicting Riolan's findings and not merely questioning them.

It is probable that Harvey's very first demonstrations were to the members of the College only, and private. But he does say 'in my anatomical lectures' *in praelectionibus meis Anatomicis*, and this has been taken to mean that he first revealed the circulation of the blood during the course of a public anatomy. Though it is difficult to ascertain precisely from the records still preserved by the College in which years Harvey did hold a general public anatomy, there is some reason to suggest that he did so every year between 1620 and 1627, with the exception of 1621 and 1625. The only independent witness of these lectures so far known is Sir Simonds D'Ewes, who attended them for three days in March 1623. Unfortunately, he merely says that he 'gained much profitable knowledge' by his attendance and makes no mention of the topics discussed. But as attendance at these public anatomies was obligatory for Candidates, Licenciates and even Fellows, it is strange that if Harvey really did discuss the circulation of the blood at any of these formal anatomies, no one is known to have referred to his new theory. During the relevant period, Thomas Moundeford, Henry Atkins and Sir William Paddy were all Presidents of the College. Among the Fellows who could have attended were Harvey's contemporaries and friends, Simon Fox and Matthew Lister, both of whom had been with him in Padua, Robert Fludd and Richard Andrews, whom Harvey named to deputise for him at St Bartholomew's Hospital, to say nothing of Sir Matthew Gwynne, Otwell Meverell, Paul de Laune, Helkiah Crooke and Theodore Goulston. Among the younger generation, Alexander Read and Francis Prujean were both Candidates and could certainly have seen Harvey's demonstrations, but if they did, neither they nor anyone else so far known has admitted to it. Yet the public announcement of the circulation of the blood must have made a ripple on the pond, even if it only gave rise to expressions of doubt and scepticism and did not provoke an immediate outcry of ridicule and downright denial. So we come to the suggestion that whatever Harvey means by the reference to his 'anatomical lectures', he does not mean that it was during the formal public anatomies given in the College that he first demonstrated the circulation of the blood.

In support of this hypothesis there are various considerations, in addition to the strange lack of any reference to this even on the part of any of those who, we may be certain, attended. As has been said, the purpose of these formal anatomies was to teach the basic essentials of anatomy. They were not the occasion for the discussion of new or controversial subjects. There was not time in the course of three days to enter into any topic of anatomical controversy. Moreover, if much of the audience had not yet learnt the grammar and vocabulary of the subject, they could not be expected to understand the fruits of the latest research. Further to this point, these formal anatomies were conducted on one or more cadavers. It is not possible to demonstrate the circulation of the blood in a cadaver. It can be explained and described, but it cannot be shown. To show it taking place, Harvey must have used living animals. We know that in Bologna in 1540, Vesalius used living dogs in the course of his anatomical demonstrations. We know that at Padua a variety of animals was used by Fabricius for teaching anatomy, including in 1584, a living gravid ewe. We know that after 1660, experiments on living animals were performed before the Royal Society meeting at Gresham College. But there is no evidence to lead us to suppose that living animals were used, either at the hall of the Barber-Surgeons or at the College of Physicians, on the occasions of the formal anatomies held in those institutions during the first half of the seventeenth century. Hogarth's drawing, The Reward of Cruelty, which depicts an anatomy in progress at the College of Physicians, does show a dog sniffing the entrails, but the date is 1750 and it would be wrong to lay too much emphasis on the evidence of this picture. Nowhere in the records of either the Physicians or the Barber-Surgeons is there any reference to the use of animals. We know nothing about the manner in which anatomies were conducted at the College of Physicians, but we do know of the ceremony attendant on the formal anatomy held at the Barber-Surgeons. We know of the mat to be provided for the lecturer's feet lest he took cold, of the two fine white rods with which he was to demonstrate the parts, of the wax candle to let him look inside the body, of the aprons, from the shoulder downwards, and the clean sleeves which he was to be given to wear. We know of the steps taken to procure the bodies and the difficulties experienced. If animals had been used, some mention at least might have been made of them. It is not to be supposed that the Lumleian anatomies at the College of Physicians, or the College's own annual anatomy were occasions for less ceremony or were conducted in any manner differently from those held by the Barber-Surgeons. That being so, and in view of the improbability that living animals were used, all that Harvey could have done at a formal anatomy was to show the structure of the valves of the veins from the cadaver and demonstrate their use on the ligated arm of a bystander, in the manner he describes in De motu cordis. But as this kind of demonstration was used by Fabricius in Padua to a totally different purpose, we may well wonder whether this in itself would have been sufficient to convince an audience of uninitiated of the truth of the hypothesis of the circulation, without all the supporting evidence which Harvey provides in his book.

Another point that makes one wonder whether Harvey really demonstrated the circulation at the formal anatomies is the text of the Lectures themselves. If Harvey used this manuscript, as the additions to it imply, up to at least 1626, we may well ask why it contains no references to the crucial experiments by which the circulation was proved and why all the statements which are inconsistent with the hypothesis of the circulation are left uncorrected. If he had indeed referred to the circulation in the Lectures, it is not unreasonable to suppose that some trace of it at least might have been found in the manuscript. The point is all the more relevant from the fact that these notes do contain his observations on the movement of the heart, its ventricles and auricles, on the movement of the blood in the arteries and his experiments and arguments by which he proved that systole and diastole were the reverse of what was generally supposed. If we now turn to Harvey's other reference in *De motu cordis*, cap. 1, to his 'Anatomy Lectures', it is plain that it is to this demonstration that he is alluding. Having recounted the difficulties he experienced in observing the movement of the heart when he first began, and having explained that only by 'using daily more search and diligence' did he finally think that he had 'gain'd both the motion and use of the heart, together with that of the arteries', he adds:

> Since which time I have not been afraid, both privately to my friends, and publickly in my Anatomy Lectures to deliver my opinion (p. 17).

By 1616, Harvey's observations on the heart's movements were sufficiently advanced for him to be certain that what he had to say on the subject was true, for he is hardly likely to have invited his audience to share his bewilderment. I would, therefore, suggest that both the references to the Anatomy Lectures may allude to the discussion of the heart's movement and his new theory concerning systole and diastole, and not to any discussion of the circulation of the blood throughout the whole body. This hypothesis would fit the facts as they are at present known. The announcement of the circulation of the blood at a public anatomy did not make a stir, because it was not then announced. Harvey did not have the problem of deciding how to fit it in to the compass of a three-day anatomy, or how to explain it to those who did not yet know enough about accepted theory to understand the force of his arguments refuting it. The notes for the Lectures do not conceal what he said, but reveal it. They do not constitute Harvey's experimental notebook, but show that, like Galileo, he continued to teach in accordance with the best authorities of his day at a time when he was beginning to realise, and ultimately to know, that some of these opinions were false. They have nothing to do with Harvey's demonstrations to the members of the College of Physicians of the circulation of the blood. With one exception, they afford no help with the problem of how his ideas developed or what experiments he performed and in what order. The exception is the reference made to Riolan in 1626, where the query would seem to imply that this was a fact new to Harvey and one which he had not then verified experimentally, but his knowledge of the valves of the veins lead him to expect the reverse of Riolan's findings.

In 1627, Harvey was writing notes for a treatise he never published, *De motu locali animalium*. All the evidence seems to show that by then he must have completed his work on the circulation, yet it affords no help in clarifying his state of mind. Much of the work relates to Aristotle's writings on the movement of animals and to Fabricius's treatises on the movement of muscles and joints. In it Harvey alludes several times to the movement of the heart, but all his remarks amount to nothing more than the statement that its movement is beyond the control of the will and the speculation that its motive power is occasioned by the spirit:

> By the spirit is occasioned the beating of the heart, Δ the right ventricle pulsates last and in the foetus the punctum saliens always pulsates[2] (p. 95).

There are three references to *De motu cordis*, but each is an addition to the text. The first merely says 'See the book *De motu cordis*' and replaces a passage on the classification of movement into animal, natural and vital, which has been crossed out (p. 21). The second says 'See *De motu cordis* as to whether there is movement of the vital spirit' (p. 45) and may be taken to refer to cap. 15. The third, 'The extent of the action can be commensurate with the whole body, see WH's book' (p. 49), is presumably an allusion to his statement in *De motu cordis*, cap. 9, that the blood is impelled by the arterial pulse through every part and member of the body in an incessant stream.

Harvey himself says that he solved the problem of the movement of the blood by having frequent recourse to vivisections, by employing a variety of animals and by collecting numerous observations. At some stage these observations ceased to be random. Though numerous observations on a variety of animals will be found in his Lectures of 1616, showing that this habit of work was already his, yet these observations are not guided in any particular direction and only some of those which were necessary for *De motu cordis* had been made. It is his animal experiments which are lacking in the Lectures. He refers to the vivisection of a dog which he had performed for the purpose of inspecting its thymus, and that his observations on the movement of the heart had been carried out on living animals is plain. In fact he says of his conclusion on the arterial pulse: 'This can be proved by actual inspection in the living and in the dead' (p. 269). But apart from making an incision in the ventricle and watching the blood spurt out at each contraction, he mentions no other experiments on a living animal. In *De motu locali animalium*, he alludes to the fact that a frog moves after its heart has been excised, and possibly to the movements of an eel in the same condition. But these experiments he had already performed by 1616, for in the Lectures he says, 'After the heart has been cut out, a frog skips, an eel crawls and a dog walks' (p. 253). Moreover, these experiments are not so much concerned with his work on the heart as with his study of nerves and of the part which they play in movement. That Harvey had consummate skill in dissection and vivisection is unquestionable, and in this context it is worth noting his reference in *De motu locali animalium* to an experiment involving artificial ventilation, a technique which, when it was demonstrated to the Fellows of the Royal Society by Robert Hooke in 1667, seems to have been considered a novelty: 'A cock's head off, the arteries being tied and artificial ventilation given (*respirationi dato loco*), movements are seen to persist . . .' etc. (p. 103). Though not an experiment connected with the movement of the heart or blood, it proves that in 1627 Harvey was in possession of a technique by which he could perform all the necessary animal experiments for the purpose of proving his hypothesis of the circulation.

Before 1628, and perhaps before 1625, Harvey had to perform all the experiments recorded in *De motu cordis*: dividing the arteries in dogs, dividing the veins, and in both cases watching and assessing the results; tying the veins in snakes and fish below the heart and watching the space between the ligature and the heart become empty of blood; watching the blood spurt from the proximal side of a cut artery and from the distal side of a severed vein. All these experiments are of the utmost elegance and simplicity and they would not have taken long to perform, but each must have been repeated again and again until Harvey was sufficiently satisfied of the truth of his new hypothesis, that the blood circulated throughout the whole body, to be ready to publish it to the world.

NOTES

1. It has not escaped the attention of various critics in the past that 'nine years and more' is the ideal period advocated by Horace for the maturing of a literary work. They have, therefore, tended to regard this phrase as meaning merely 'a long time'. It was a convenient interpretation while it was still believed that in 1616 Harvey first discussed the circulation of the blood in his Lumleian lectures, for it explained away the twelve years which actually elapsed between the lectures and the publication of *De motu cordis*. The literal interpretation of Harvey's words now seems to fit the facts.

2. As is well known, Harvey uses the sign Δ with the meaning 'it may be shown' possibly as an abbreviation for 'demonstrandum'.

Chapter Six

De Motu Cordis *1628*

IN the autumn of 1628, a small and modest-looking book was published in Leyden. Surprise has sometimes been expressed as to why Harvey should have chosen to send his manuscript to Holland, but the reason is an obvious one. At that date the three great centres for the publication of medical and scientific works were Frankfurt, Venice and Leyden. Books appearing from the presses of these cities were certain to be noticed by the universities of Europe, which was not necessarily the case with works published in the British Isles. If, moreover, as has been suggested, Harvey's friend Robert Fludd knew the printer William Fitzer, Harvey's choice of Leyden is easy to understand.

Much has been said about the rare excellence of *De motu cordis* and it is doubtful whether anything more could be usefully added. It will be sufficient, therefore, if we try to discover whether it affords any clue as to the stages by which Harvey's thought developed. We can accordingly delay consideration of the Introductory chapter until later, for this can only have been written once Harvey's new hypothesis was not only postulated but proved experimentally.

The first seven chapters contain observations and experiments many of which Harvey had already recorded in 1616. It would seem obvious, therefore, that his attack on the whole problem began from the work which he did in the testing of the hypothesis of Columbus concerning systole and diastole of the heart. It is also certain that when he began this work he had no idea of the conclusion to which he would in-exorably be led. Even when this work was completed, the hypothesis of the circulation of the blood had not been formulated. That came later. If, as he told Robert Boyle, it was the consideration of the valves in the veins that first gave him a clue, the work in connection with these must have come first. What came next would seem to have been the question of the amount of blood extruded by the heart at each beat. If the hypothesis was then formulated, it is possible that at this stage he saw the important experimental proof which could be provided by the ligatures of varying tightness around the arm. On these two questions, the action of the valves of the veins and the quantity of blood in the body, rests the whole hypothesis of the circulation. And it may be that this is the order in which the problem was unravelled.

The first chapter contains nothing to the purpose, for it is merely Harvey's account of his reasons for writing the book. It also says, as we have already seen, that he had demonstrated his new theories on systole and diastole of the heart during the course of his Anatomical Lectures. He begins the attack on systole and diastole of the heart in cap. 2. Here there are no new observations, new that is since 1616, but, as one might expect, confirmation of the fact that they have been made over and over again during the course of the intervening years. Harvey stresses here the obvious importance of observing the heart's movement in cold-blooded animals, and the list which he gives is far longer than in his Lectures: toads, frogs, snakes, small fish, crabs, shrimps, shell-fish and snails. He also speaks of watching the heart as its movements begin to flag in dying dogs and pigs. The four points which he then makes will all be found in the Lectures, though not arranged with equal cogency.

> So then these things happen at one and the same time, the tension of the heart, the erection of the point, the beating (which is felt outwardly by reason of its hitting against the breast), the incrassation of the sides of it, and the forcible protrusion of the blood by constriction of the ventricles. Hence the contrary of the commonly received opinion appears. . . . For that motion which is commonly thought the Diastole of the heart, is really the Systole, and so the proper motion of the heart is not Diastole but a Systole, for the heart receives no vigour in the Diastole, but in the Systole, for then it is extended, moveth, and receiveth vigour (pp. 21–2).

Harvey concludes the chapter with a reasoned disagreement with Vesalius's analysis of the movement of the heart in terms of the alternate contraction of its longitudinal and transverse fibres, and his analogy with a bunch of rushes.[1] As we have already seen, Harvey makes his point here clearly and vigorously from the knowledge he has gained from his work on muscular contraction in general. He disposes once and for all of this erroneous notion which, because it was associated with the name of Vesalius, had won for itself considerable acceptance. As a tail-piece to the chapter, Harvey denies the attractive power of the heart, the erroneous notion which seems to underlie Vesalius's erroneous explanation of the heart's movement. But Harvey leaves the discussion of how the heart does receive the blood until later. It was an explanation which followed once the hypothesis of the circulation had been made.

Cap. 3 is devoted to the movement of the arteries, and here again most of the observations had already been recorded in the Lectures. Only one or two points call for comment. As before, it is obvious that Harvey has observed the movement of the arteries in many more experiments on living animals, and certain refinements consequent upon this are added to the basic remarks made in the Lectures. These refinements relate to the cessation of the arterial pulse when the ventricles cease to contract, and to the possibility of interfering with it by compression. It was perhaps due to the fortunate chance that delivered into his hands a patient with a large aneurysm that led him to make these further experimental observations. He has also noticed that the size of the pulse varies with the size of the heart-beat, and it may have been this which first gave him the idea of estimating the total amount of blood in the body. Another observation concerns the pulmonary artery, whose pulsation he notes is contemporaneous with the contraction of the right ventricle and ceases when the right ventricle ceases to pulsate. There is no doubt that he was pleased to find corroboration for his views in Aristotle. Harvey then concludes:

> Wherefore, whether it be by compression, stuffing (sc. infarction), or interception that the motion of the blood through the arteries be hindered, in that case the furthermost arteries do beat less, seeing the pulse of the arteries is nothing but the impulsion of blood into the arteries (p. 27).

In the next chapter, Harvey analyses the movement of the auricles. The first thing to notice here is the new experiment which he has performed. In the Lectures he merely says that the blood is driven into the ventricles by the contraction of the auricles, but cites no experiment in proof.

> But this is chiefly to be observed, that after the heart has left beating and the ears are beating still, putting your finger upon the ventricle of the heart, every pulsation is perceived in the ventricles, just after the same manner as we said the pulsations of the ventricles were felt in the Arteries, a distension being made by impulsion of blood: and at the same

time, the ears only beating, if you cut away the point of the heart with a pair of Scissors, you shall see the blood flow from thence at every pulsation of the ear, so that from thence it appears which way the blood comes into the ventricles, not by attraction or distension of the heart, but sent in by the impulsion of the ears (p. 29).

The further work which he has done on the auricles enables him to analyse the movement of the heart as consisting of four motions distinct in place but not in time, for the two auricles move simultaneously and then the two ventricles, and so he contradicts politely the findings of both Bauhin and Riolan. It has also led him to a more precise description of the action of the auricles in a dying heart, and to the observation that in this condition the ventricles respond only after two or more auricular beats. This is perhaps one of the finest pieces of observation and description in the whole of *De motu cordis*.

> When all things are already in a languishing condition, (the heart dying away, as it is both in Fishes and other colder animals which have blood) there intercedes some short resting time betwixt these two motions, and the heart being as it were weakened, seems to answer the motion, sometimes swifter, sometimes slower; last of all drawing towards death, it ceases to answer by its motion, and only by nodding its head seems to give consent, and moves so insensibly, that it seems only to give a sign of motion to the ears: So the heart first leaves beating before the ears, so that the ears are said to out-live it: the left ventricle leaves beating first of all, then its ear, then the right ventricle, last of all (which Galen observes) all the rest giving off and dying, the right ear beats still: so that life seems to remain last of all in the right. And whilst by little and little the heart is dying, you may see after two or three beatings of the ear, the heart will, being as it were rowsed, answer, and very slowly and hardly [*sc.* reluctantly, or with difficulty] endeavour and frame a motion (pp. 28–9).

In addition to the points which it has in common with the Lectures, this chapter contains nothing that is directly relevant to the hypothesis which Harvey will presently propound. What is included is concerned with his work on the generation of animals and his speculations on the life which appears to be inherent in the blood. Their discussion will be for the moment deferred.

All the points which Harvey has so far made are thus seen to be either observations collected before 1616 or more observations on the same things. Cap. 5 is different. It is a summary, made with consummate skill and not a little artistry, of the preceding chapters, and concerns 'The action and the office of the motions of the Heart'. Needless to say, the description of the action is more vivid and more graphic than anything written in 1616, for it is here that Harvey compares the rhythmical movement of the auricles and ventricles to firing a shot and to the action of swallowing. The reflection that the alternate movements of the auricles and ventricles keep 'a certain harmony and number' is a reminder of the fact that in *De motu locali animalium* Harvey had spent some time in thinking about the harmony and rhythm of muscular action and so of the different movements of the body. When describing how a horse drinks and swallows, Harvey notices that the movement of the throat can be both heard and felt; in the same way a pulse can be heard in the chest when the heart transmits the blood from the veins to the arteries.[2] Harvey concludes this part of the chapter with the promise to discuss later whether or not the heart transmits anything more than blood, that is to say heat, spirit or perfection.

On balance it would seem that by 1616 Harvey had accepted the truth of Columbus's findings concerning the pulmonary transit of the blood, based as it was on the understanding of the competence of the valves of the heart and the non-porosity of the ventricular septum. If it could be granted that transfusion of blood from the arteries to the veins occurred in the lungs – and the parallel adduced with the transfusion of blood in the liver was accepted as convincing – then there was no need of further experiments to prove this point. Consequently Harvey may have left the further elaboration of this subject until after his work on the valves of the veins had led him to formulate the hypothesis of the circulation throughout the body. The question of the competence of the valves of the veins and of the valves of the heart is obviously linked, and after satisfying himself on the competence of the valves of the veins, it is possible that Harvey returned to the problem of the pulmonary transit of the blood, a phenomenon which at the time was still not generally accepted. Knowing that the hypothesis of ventricular pores was totally unnecessary, Harvey had to suggest the existence of an alternative pathway by which the blood from the right ventricle could reach the left. The alternative pathway was ready to hand in animals with no lungs and in the foetus. Consequently, the second part of this chapter is forward looking and logical rather than chronological in order. From the standpoint of his greater knowledge he can survey the cause of error and realise that it had arisen from the intimate anatomical connection that exists in man between the heart and the lungs. From this had come the belief that respiration, the essential action of the lungs, and the movement of the heart served the same purpose. Because of this, all the anatomists were stumbling in the dark. As Harvey himself had been in that position in 1616, this realisation can only have come after the knowledge that the blood did circulate throughout the body, and that the movement of the heart was designed to propel the blood and was utterly unconnected with the movement of the lungs. It is to prove this point that his work on animals with no lungs and on the foetus was undertaken. The second part of this chapter, then, forms a bridge leading from one subject to the next.

Courteously assuming that all anatomists really agree with his account of the heart's movements thus far (his polite optimism is more than apparent from the writing of his contemporaries), he says that from here on,

> stumbling as it were in a dark place, they seem to be dim-sighted, and clamper up divers things, which are contrary and inconsistent, and speak many things at random. . . . One thing seems to me to have been the chief cause of doubt and mistake in this business, which is, the contexture [*sc.* intimate connection] in man of the heart and lungs; For when they did see the *vena arteriosa*, and the *arteria venosa*, coming likewise into the lungs, and there to disappear, it could not sink with them [*sc.* they were much at a loss to see] either how the right ventricle should distribute the blood into the body, or how the left ventricle should draw it out of the *vena Cava* (pp. 37–8).

The references which Harvey then proceeds to make to Galen's refutation of Erasistratus doubtless illuminated the subject for his contemporaries, and had the advantage of allowing him to claim that, in some sort, his opinion had the authority of Galen to support it. His intention is to prove that the aorta in fact distributes the blood throughout the whole body and for this he claims Galen's support. Galen had refuted the belief that air was present in the arteries, thereby upsetting the neat system of Erasistratus according to which the veins contained blood and the arteries air and the two sets of vessels did not communicate. When Galen showed that there was blood and not air in the arteries, the problem was to explain how it got there: hence the invention of the invisible pores in the septum and the anastomoses between veins and arteries. Otherwise the anatomists could not explain the presence after death in the left ventricle of the heart and in the pulmonary vein of the 'thick, knotty, black blood'. Harvey is not here concerned to prove that the septum is a solid wall, but to show that there is an alternative pathway and consequently no need to assume the existence of pores. He was evidently convinced by his own findings that these pores did not exist, and, confident in the knowledge that Vesalius and other anatomists agreed with him, did not think experimental proof necessary. So here, remarking that he has already 'refuted' this notion, he passes on to the discussion in the next chapter of the alternative pathway by which the blood is transmitted from the veins to the arteries. If for a moment we turn back to his 'refutation', which will be found in the Introductory chapter, it will be seen that it consists merely in a flat denial:

> By my troth there are no such pores, nor can any be demonstrated. For the substance of the septum of the heart is thicker and more compact, than any part of the body, except the bones and nerves (p. 13).

That he denied the existence of pores already in 1616 has been noticed, although Bauhin's findings in the ox's heart remained inexplicable. As there is no mention of it here, he had probably dismissed it as an anomaly. Because he gave no experimental proof of the impermeability of the septum, deeming it unnecessary, this was one of the points seized upon by his critics in their efforts to bring down his whole theory.

There is considerable doubt as to whether Harvey had realised in 1616 the importance which he would come to attach to his observations on animals having hearts with only one ventricle, and on the foetal heart. The problem is closely linked with that of the pulmonary transit of the blood and, as we know that this was already in his mind by 1616, we will assume that cap. 7 of De motu cordis chronologically precedes cap. 6 and discuss it first.

From the point of view of experimental evidence it is a singularly disappointing chapter. Harvey has performed no new experiments but lets it be inferred that he has repeated the observations made by Columbus in the course of vivisections, and probably that he has also repeated his simple experiments. What he has to say is not so much a demonstration of the truth of the phenomenon as an impassioned appeal for belief in what Columbus had said. Since no difficulty seems to be encountered in believing that blood percolates through the parenchyma of the liver,

> Why should they not likewise believe this of the passage of the blood through the lungs in men come to age, upon the same arguments? And

with Columbus, a most skilfull and learned Anatomist, believe and assert the same from the structure and largeness of the lungs; because the *Arteria venosa* [*sc.* pulmonary vein], and likewise the ventricle, are always full of blood, which must needs come hither out of the veins by no other path but through the lungs; as both he and we from our words before, our own eye-sight, and other Arguments, do believe to be clear (pp. 50–1).

The chapter is in effect devoted to an attempt to win belief for the percolation of the blood through the parenchyma of the lungs by means of various analogies: water percolating through the earth gives rise to springs and fountains, sweat passes through the skin, urine through the parenchyma of the kidneys.[3] On this last point he adds various observations, also to be found in the Lectures, by way of strengthening the analogy. So he falls to upbraiding the unbelievers and points out that it is more difficult to believe that blood percolates through the parenchyma of the liver than through that of either the kidneys or the lungs. For its flesh is denser, it has no impulsive force to drive the blood and it is not, like the lungs, perpetually in motion. As everyone agrees that the 'juyce of all things we receive' passes through the liver, why not admit that the whole mass of blood permeates the substance of the lungs in the same way.[4] At this juncture, instead of devising experiments to demonstrate the competence of the valves of the heart, Harvey falls back on the opinions of Galen whom he proceeds to quote at length, 'seeing there are some such persons which admit nothing, unless there be an authority alleged for it'. Whether the passages quoted from Galen actually mean what Harvey intends them to is another matter. With a little judicious alteration and interpretation he can make them fit his purpose well enough. Then and only then, does he explain why he is convinced of the truth of the hypothesis:

Furthermore it was necessary that the heart should receive the blood continually into the ventricles as in a pond or cistern, and send it forth again: and for this reason it was necessary that it should be serv'd with four locks or doors, whereof two should serve for the intromission and two for the emission of blood, lest either the blood like an *Euripus* should inconveniently be driven up and down, or go back thither from whence it were fitter to be drawn, and flow from that part to which it was needful it should have been sent, and so be wearied with idle travel and the breathing of the lungs be hindered. Lastly our assertion appears clearly to be true, that the blood does continually and incessantly flow through the porosities of the lungs, out of the right ventricle into the left, out of the *vena cava* into the *arteria magna*; for seeing the blood is continually sent out of the right ventricle into the lungs through the *vena arteriosa* [*sc.* pulmonary artery], and likewise is continually attracted[5] out of the lungs into the left, which appears by that which has been spoken, and the position of the Portals, it cannot be, but that it must need pass through continually.

And likewise, seeing that always, and without intermission, the blood enters the right ventricle of the heart, and goes out (which is likewise manifest of the left ventricle, both by reason and sense), it is impossible but that the blood should pass continually through, out of the *vena cava* into the Aorta (pp. 54-5).

The appeal for men to believe in what they see recalls Columbus's similar and even more impassioned plea on this very point. Perhaps it is not too wide of the mark to suggest that Harvey's demonstrations or discussions of the pulmonary transit of the blood during his anatomies, or with members of the College of Physicians, had met with obstinate refusal to be convinced. Harvey ends the chapter by referring to what happens in animals with only one ventricle and no lungs, and adds that when Nature wanted to send the blood through the lungs, she added the right ventricle for this very purpose.[6]

During his investigation of the arterial pulse and its connection with the heart beat, Harvey had evidently performed an experiment on a fish, cutting the ventral aorta and watching the blood spurt out at each contraction of the heart. He had already noticed in 1616 that the 'bladder of blood' at the base of the heart served the office of an auricle. The experiment and the observation were both of use in cap. 6, for they allowed him to state that in all animals of this kind it is obvious that the blood passes directly from the veins into the heart and from the heart into the arteries, obvious, that is to say, to anyone who will dissect a live fish and look. He says the same for animals in which the lungs exist but are far removed from the heart, and incidentally alludes to the fact that he had collected many observations on the lungs of different animals.[7] As Harvey is really only concerned to prove here that blood goes from the veins to the arteries without going through the septum of the heart, he has made his point.

The logical transition from the study of animals with no lungs to man goes by way of the foetal heart. At this time the anatomical structure of the vessels of the foetal heart was more or less correctly known; it was their interpretation which was at fault. It will be remembered that according to the traditional account, the blood from the vena cava, instead of going into the right ventricle, was sent directly through a pore or an anastomosis (the foramen ovale, but not so called) into the pulmonary vein and from thence into the lungs to supply them with natural blood for their nourishment. The foramen ovale was covered by a large membrane, or 'lid', which allowed the passage of the blood into the pulmonary vein, but prevented its regurgitation into the vena cava. The canal or pipe (Harvey calls it the 'second aorta' and it is of course the ductus arteriosus), which linked the aorta and pulmonary artery, was thought to supply the lungs with vital blood. As the aorta is set higher than the pulmonary artery, it was held that the blood could easily run downhill into it, and there were no valves at the base of the aorta to prevent it. (What happened when the foetus moved around and turned head down does not seem to have crossed their minds.) At this point it had to be explained that the pulmonary vein, for them the venous artery, served in the foetus the office of a vein, and contrariwise, the pulmonary artery, their arterial vein, that of an artery. In addition, it was believed that the foetal heart did not beat, and that both the venous and arterial blood derived directly from the mother through the umbilical veins and arteries and ebbed and flowed backwards and forwards to the maternal heart. Venous and arterial blood were supplied to the heart through the coronary veins and arteries, thus providing it with the means to exist. This system did not allow for the presence of any blood in the right ventricle of the foetal heart, and this was thought to be correct because, as the heart did not move, if there were any, it would stagnate. Nor was there any spirit in the left ventricle. The foetus thus seems to have been considered in every sense a passenger and a parasite.

Harvey reasonably objects to the belief that the purpose of the union of the vessels is the nourishment of the lungs, seeing that their blood supply would thus be greater in the foetus, when they are inactive, than in the adult, when they are in use. It is, as he says, 'improbable and inconsistent'. He further terms 'false' the notion that the foetal heart does not beat, for he has proved the contrary by many inspections and can cite Aristotle's opinion in his support. But Harvey is not here concerned with a general attack on the foetal circulation. He is merely using the foetal heart as a further proof of his contention that the blood is propelled from the vena cava into the aorta 'by as open ways as if both the ventricles . . . were made pervious to one another, by taking away the portion betwixt them' (p. 47). He is content for this purpose to take over and incorporate as part of his text, the description of the foramen ovale verbatim from the textbook of Bauhin, merely changing the end of one sentence. Instead of saying with Bauhin that the blood passes through the foramen ovale out of the vena cava into the pulmonary artery 'and so is carried to the lungs', he substitutes, into the pulmonary artery 'and the left ear of the heart', and so to the left ventricle (p. 43). His description of the ductus arteriosus is likewise basically not his own but comes from the same source. His conclusion as to its use, however, is his own and correct.

> So that here we have reason to think [i.e. because of the valves at the base of the pulmonary artery], that in an Embryon when the heart contracts itself, the blood must always be carried out of the right ventricle into the *arteria magna* by this way (p. 45).

Harvey's conclusion, therefore, which he has reached by many inspections of living foetuses rather than by any experiment, is that the blood passes from the vena cava through the foramen ovale into the pulmonary vein, the left auricle and left ventricle, from whence, when the heart contracts, it is driven into the aorta. The right ventricle also receives blood from the right auricle and from the vena cava, and when the heart contracts this blood is driven through the ductus arteriosus into the aorta. With the rest of the difficulties in the traditional account of the movement of the blood in the foetus, Harvey is not concerned, and they are not discussed. He has proved his point and brought the blood from the right side of the heart to the left by obvious and patent ways. If at birth these passages are closed, and instead the way is opened to the lungs, then through the lungs the blood must go in the adult from the right to the left ventricle.

> So then the business is arriv'd to this, that to those who search for the veins in man (by which the blood passes out of the *vena cava* into the left ventricle and into the *arteria venosa*) it were more worthy their pains, and wiselier done, if from the dissection of living creatures they would search the truth, why in the greater and more perfect creatures, and those of riper age, nature would rather have the blood squeezed through the streyner of the lungs, than through the most patent passages, as in other creatures: and then they would understand that no other way nor passage could be excogitated (pp. 47–8).

With a sidelong glance at the reason, that the lungs may cool the blood, and a promise to discuss it further on some other occasion, Harvey leaves the subject.

Cap. 8, 'Of the abundance of blood passing through the Heart out of the veins into the arteries, and of the circular motion of the blood', occupies the central position in the book. Everything that has so far been said looks forward to it; everything that follows looks back to it. It is the climax and the crisis of the work. The symmetry is unlikely to have been fortuitous. Within the chapter itself there is a similar symmetry. It consists of nine different points, of which the fifth, in the very centre, is the announcement of the hypothesis. The first four prepare for it, the last four surround it. Harvey begins by saying that everything that has so far been discussed, is more or less in accordance with the teaching of Galen and Columbus, and will doubtless command agreement. What remains to be said is novel. Consequently, he fears the enmity of mankind, but in spite of this must proceed. He surveys the evidence which he has accumulated. This evidence suggests the circular movement of the blood which he then propounds. He seeks an analogy from Aristotle and applies the analogy to the movement of the blood. He praises the heart. He concludes by pointing to the difference between veins and arteries. It is of the greatest importance to notice precisely what Harvey says of the formulation of the hypothesis, and this because it has been suggested that Harvey was much influenced by the philosophy of circles current among the more esoteric thinkers of his day, and that he thought first of the circle and then of the facts. Harvey's own words refute this notion, for he makes it abundantly plain that the facts which he had accumulated imposed the circular notion of the flow of blood on his conclusion.

> Truly when I had often and seriously considered with myself, what great abundance there was, both by the dissection of living things, for experiment's sake, and the opening of arteries, and many ways of searching, and from the Symetrie and magnitude of the ventricles of the heart, and of the vessels which go into it, and go out from it, (since Nature, making nothing in vain, did not allot that greatness proportionably to no purpose, to those vessels) as likewise from the continued and careful artifice of the doores and fibers, and the rest of the fabrick, and from many other things; and when I had a long time considered with myself how great abundance of blood was passed through, and in how short time that transmission was done, whether or no the juyce of the nourishment which

we receive could furnish this or no: at last I perceived that the veins should be quite emptied, and the arteries on the other side be burst with too much intrusion of blood, unless the blood did pass back again some way out of the veins into the arteries and return into the right ventricle of the heart.

I began to bethink myself if it might not have a circular motion . . . (pp 57–8).

No plainer statement of the way in which the hypothesis was reached could be desired. So all scientific discovery is made. First comes the uneasy feeling that something is wrong with accepted theory, that there is some dissonance which breaks the harmony. Then follows the search for more and new facts. A temporary hypothesis is made; experiments designed to test it; and this not once but many times. So little by little the facts, demonstrable to the senses in the seventeenth-century phrase, are accumulated and then, and only then, comes the postulating of an hypothesis which seems to account for every known fact and which is dictated by the facts themselves. After that follow more experiments designed to test its truth. This process is sometimes called the 'hypothetico-deductive' method. It is the method used by the modern biologist. It was the method used by Harvey. On its foundation in 1660, the Royal Society laid down as one of its basic tenets that nothing was to be accepted 'on any man's word', *nullius in verba*. By so doing it gave formal expression to an idea which had been growing more common during the preceding half-century. Harvey accepts nothing on the authority of his predecessors, Aristotle, Galen or any man. But he shows himself different from the modern biologist in that, having found incontrovertible experimental proof of his hypothesis, he turns to the past in search of some statement which he can cite in support of his theory. It is apparently for this reason that he quotes at this point the cosmic analogy of Aristotle:

> Which motion we may call circular, after the same manner that *Aristotle* sayes that the rain and air do imitate the motion of the superior bodies. For the earth being wet, evaporates by the heat of the Sun, and the vapours being rais'd aloft are condens'd and descend in showrs and wet the ground . . . (p. 59).

It could be argued that Aristotle's analogy is a bad one for only by a feat of the imagination can the circular motion of the heavens, that is, the eternal revolution of the heavenly bodies and spheres around the earth, be compared with the eternal ascent and descent of vapour and rain. The only point they have in common is their eternity, and for Aristotle it was axiomatic that all eternal motion was circular. Hence the analogy and its inherent discrepancy. For Harvey the choice of the analogy was indicated, as he explains in the next paragraph, by speculation based on physiological observation combined with acceptance, in this context, of Aristotle's opinion on the primacy of the heart. Without the heart there could be no circulation of blood; this was a physiological fact. But the heart had acquired what one might call its own mythology. Its importance in the body had been recognised for generations before any idea of its true function could be had. It was variously described as the seat of the soul, of the spirit, of the intelligence, of the emotions and passions, and this over and above the Aristotelian opinions of more physiological flavour by which it was regarded as the source of vital heat in the body, as that without which nothing in the body could exist. For generations it had been compared with the sun and the comparison is a very obvious one. Harvey knew experimentally that when an artery is occluded, the parts beyond the ligature grow cold. What more natural than that he should assume with Aristotle that the heart imparts warmth from its own vital heat to the blood returning from the members before sending it again upon its course. Hence the relevance of the analogy with the vapours and the rain. It was not Harvey's fault that this led some of his contemporaries into error. This same analogy had already been used by alchemists and some esoteric philosophers to describe the process of distillation, a fundamental process in alchemy. Consequently, this process acquired from the analogy the name 'circulation', a misnomer, for it is ascent and descent which is implied, not going around. Harvey by circulation means first and foremost a going around. The ideas of ascent and descent are only introduced in an attempt to reconcile his fundamental concept with an unfortunate analogy of Aristotle. That it did lead to some confusion is proved by the fact that Sir George Ent changed the title of his *Apologia* from *pro circulatione sanguinis* as it had appeared in the first edition of 1641, to *pro circuitione sanguinis* in the second edition of 1685, thus avoiding the use of this 'technical term' and putting his meaning beyond any possible doubt. As Ent was a friend of Harvey, we may accept this as conclusive evidence of the meaning attached by Harvey himself to the word 'circulation'. As has already been said, it has nothing to do with the meaning attached to it by Caesalpinus or by Paracelsus and his followers.

127

Harvey's own words leave no room for doubt that it was the facts assembled before him that dictated the hypothesis of circular movement, for it was the only one into which they all fitted. His approach to any problem was essentially pragmatic. 'I do not profess to learn and teach Anatomy from the axioms of the Philosophers, but from Dissections and from the fabrick of Nature' (p. xiii). Deeply read as he was in the works of Aristotle, he was of course aware of the analogy which could be drawn between the movement of the blood and the various circular motions instanced by Aristotle. But this is not to say that Aristotle's philosophy, any more than that of Paracelsus, had any part whatsoever in the formulation of the hypothesis. If this were so, one might well ask why no-one before him had reached this conclusion. The essential pieces of evidence were already to hand before Harvey gave his Lumleian lectures for the first time in 1616. Nor is it likely that it was speculation on the purpose of the blood's movement that led to the hypothesis of its circular motion. No word of this has yet been said in *De motu cordis*. Each chapter is concerned with the understanding of how various phenomena happen, not why they do. Only here, in attempting to relate Aristotle's cosmic analogy to the circulation of the blood does he for the first time suggest a reason. And it is a reason born of the belief, respectable by its ancestry, that the heart has something essential to contribute to the blood. But this he puts forward merely as a suggestion, for, as will be seen in his letter to Hofmann, he categorically denies that he had ever asserted the purpose of the circulation.[8] His views on it were in fact undecided throughout his life, but we will leave the discussion of this problem until we come to consider what he had to say on the subject in *De generatione*.[9]

The final paragraph of cap. 8 is a tail-piece in which Harvey states that the structure of veins and arteries is different because they have a different use. There is nothing new in this, only in his conclusion, that the use of the arteries is to carry blood to the parts and that of the veins to bring it back again to the heart. Though for Harvey it was axiomatic that difference in structure implied difference in use, this was not always so for his contemporaries. It seems likely that an underlying idea here is that the difference in structure depends on the difference in pressure in the blood in the vessels and so links with the notion of the heart as a muscle and with the observation that the more distal arteries appear to differ but little from veins.

It will have been noticed that among the facts which led him to the hypothesis of the circulation, Harvey makes no mention of the valves in the veins, although, if Boyle is a faithful witness, he had himself attributed to them a crucial rôle. Instead, he speaks of the great amount of the blood which passes through the heart, and how considering this led him to wonder what happened to it. The two statements do not necessarily imply a contradiction. When Harvey realised that the office of the valves of the veins was not to check the impetus of blood discharged by the heart, but completely to prevent the flow of blood away from the heart and allow it passage only in the reverse direction, and that consequently the blood in the veins moved not away from but towards the heart, this fact, coupled with his observations that the heart extruded a considerable quantity of blood at each pulsation, may have led to the dawning of the hypothesis that this blood in fact went round and back to the heart. The immediate way to test this, was to measure the total blood content of the body and the amount of blood extruded at each pulsation and find the relationship of the two to each other, and assess what this implied. And from this followed other experiments. The testimony of the valves of the veins is the crucial evidence for the return of blood to the heart. Its full weight and importance is better used when Harvey is discussing this return of the blood, and consequently it falls into the third section of the book. For the book is, after all, the logical exposition of the theory, not the chronological account of its putting together. So far Harvey has been concerned only with the movement of the heart which expels the blood into the arteries. His next logical point is the problem of what happens to the blood in the arteries and where it goes; the proof that it passes into the veins. The third and last point is the proof that it returns through the veins to the heart.

At the beginning of cap. 9, Harvey breaks down the general hypothesis of the circulation into three parts, each of which he will test by experiments designed for that purpose:

1. First, That the blood is continually, and without any intermission, transmitted out of the *vena cava* into the arteries, by the pulse of the heart, in so great abundance, that it cannot be recruited by those things we take in, and insomuch that the whole mass would quickly pass through.

2. In the second place, that continually, duly, and without cease, the blood is driven into every member and part, and enters by the pulse of the arteries, and that in far greater abundance than is necessary for nourishment, or than the whole mass is able to furnish.

   3. And likewise thirdly, that from each and every member, the veins
   themselves do perpetually bring back this blood into the mansion of
   the heart (p. 61).

Harvey began by measuring the content of the left ventricle of a man's
heart and found the answer to be something over 2oz. Estimating that
at each beat the amount extruded was between a quarter and an eighth
of the total and multiplying it by the number of beats that the heart
makes in an hour, it is immediately obvious that in a short period of
time the heart has expelled more than the total blood content of the
body. His calculations may be rough and ready, but apart from
Sanctorius,[10] a number of whose experiments were concerned with
weighing, Harvey was the first physiologist to realise the importance
which quantitative evidence could provide. His evidence is very imprecise. He did not know and could not measure the total blood content of
the human body, but he did know it and had measured it for sheep and
dogs ('for I have tryed it in a Sheep', p. 63), and the conclusion that
more blood goes through the heart than can be contained in the vessels
or produced *de novo* by the food eaten, follows from his imperfect
calculations. To the first objection, that the heart sometimes does not
propel anything, he replies that this he has refuted already, and
'besides it's against sense or reason'. Even though the amount of blood
passing out of the heart at each contraction may vary and even though
the rate at which the blood goes round the body may be different in
different circumstances, yet the least possible amount of blood expelled
into the arteries is in far greater abundance 'than it is possible that it
could be supplied by juice of nourishment which we receive, unless
there were a regress made by its circuition' (p. 65). The experience of
dissection shows that if in a living animal an artery be cut, 'all the mass
of the blood will be drain'd out of the whole body, as well out of the
veins as out of the arteries, in the space of half an hour' (ibid.). According to contemporary thinking this phenomenon could be explained
by the existence of inter-communicating anastomoses between veins
and arteries. But this, Harvey is concerned to show, is not the correct
explanation. The blood does not flow out of the veins because they
'flap down', there is no driving force in them and the valves in them
prevent anything but the smallest amount of blood being shed from
them. The arteries shed blood 'largely, impetuously, by impulsion, as
if it were cast out of a spout' (p. 66). To prove this, cut the neck artery
of a living sheep or dog and 'it will be wonderful to see, with how great

force, how great protrusion, how quickly' all the blood is emptied from veins and arteries alike. And to prove that the arteries do not receive the blood from the veins through anastomoses occurring in their course but only through the intermediary of the heart, ligate the aorta where it leaves the heart and then open the neck artery or any other artery in the body and the result will be that the arteries will empty and the veins remain full. The fact that the arteries receive blood from the veins only through the heart provides the explanation of various phenomena well known to anatomists. It explains why after death much blood is found in the veins and right ventricle and but little in the arteries and in the left ventricle. As there is no communication between veins and arteries except through the lungs and the heart, and as the lungs cease to move before the heart, the heart continues to propel the blood after supplies of blood have ceased to reach it from the lungs. It also explains why it is impossible to extract all the blood from a cadaver after the heart has ceased to beat. Harvey ends the chapter by saying that he is now trying to find the anastomoses between the veins and arteries, that no-one has described them correctly for they have all looked for them in the wrong place.

It is to be noticed that Harvey has been arguing his thesis much in the manner of any medical disputation: proposition, objection, refutation of the objection. It was the proper and approved manner of the day. Cap. 10 begins with a new objection: a cow gives milk, a woman suckles a child, and the milk is made up by the food taken in. Harvey replies that the heart sends out as much or more blood in a shorter time, thus inferring the impossibility for the digestive and concoctive organs to replace the loss so speedily. Another objection raised is that the conditions in vivisection are different from those in the intact body, and the fact that so much blood pours out of a cut artery is no proof that the like quantity goes through it normally. To this Harvey replies first by saying that the quantitative calculations prove it, and then by demonstrating it experimentally. If in a living fish or snake, the veins are ligated a little below the heart, 'you shall quickly see the distance betwixt the heart and the ligature to be emptied, so that you must needs affirm the recourse of blood, unless you will deny your own eye-sight' (p. 69).

Let us conclude, confirming all these with one example, that everyone may beleeve his own eyes: If any one cut up a live Adder, he shall see the heart beat calmly, distinctly, for a whole hour, and so contract it self (in its constriction being oblong) and thrust it self out again like a Worm. That it is whitish in the Systole, and contrary in the Diastole...(pp.69-70).

If the passage of blood through the vena cava be occluded a little below the heart, after a few beats the part of the vein between this point and the heart will be empty of blood, the heart will be whiter in colour through the lack of blood and it will beat more faintly and begin to die, but immediately the vein is untied the heart will return to its former state. Next, in the same manner, occlude the artery at a little distance from the heart. After a few beats it will swell vehemently and the heart 'beyond measure', and the heart will 'acquire a purple colour till it be blackish' and be so oppressed with blood that 'you would think it would be suffocated', but untie the artery and all will return to its former state. So there are two kinds of death, from deficiency and from excess.

Harvey proves his second contention, that the blood is driven by the heart beat into the arteries, the vessels designed to carry it away from the heart, and returns through the veins, by a series of experiments with ligatures of varying tightness described in cap. 11. If a tight ligature of the kind used for surgical operations be put round an arm, it will be noticed that the artery beyond it does not beat in the wrist or anywhere else, but above it this artery beats more vehemently and swells 'as it were with a kind of tide rise towards the ligature' (p. 74). The hand, meanwhile, retains its normal colour and only after a period of time begins to grow cold. If the ligature be then loosened till it be of middling tightness, as used in venesection, then the whole hand immediately goes red and swells almost to bursting by the force of the blood that is driven into it in ten or twelve pulsations, and he on whose arm the experiment is made will feel the warm blood entering at each arterial pulsation. If at the very moment of releasing the ligature a finger be placed on the artery, the blood will be felt passing underneath it. While the arm is still bound with a tight ligature, it will be seen that the veins above it fall away; when the ligature is loosened the veins below it become swollen and 'lumpie', so the ligature hinders the return of blood to the upper parts. Arguing from these phenomena, Harvey concludes that the blood enters the arm through the arteries; that swelling of the veins consequent upon the release of the tight ligature to middling tightness proves that the blood returns through the veins and therefore that there must be some kind of connection between the arteries and the veins at the periphery. If a small incision be made in a tiny cutaneous vein with the arm ligated for phlebotomy, all the veins which were previously lumpy will simultaneously collapse and empty themselves through the cut. The remainder of the chapter is devoted to a discussion of ligatures and what is to be understood from the expression that they 'draw'. Cap. 12 is also concerned with arguments derived from phlebotomy. As the whole blood content of the body can be emptied through a tiny incision made in a cutaneous vein in an arm ligated for phlebotomy, it follows that the arteries and the veins are connected. It is the force of the heart beat which drives the blood through the artery beyond the ligature, and the blood must have come from the vena cava into the heart and out into the artery during the actual process of the blood-letting. Turning again to the question of quantity, Harvey suggests that if the blood be allowed to flow for half an hour, the patient will be in a state near collapse because the arteries and the veins will be nearly emptied. During this period, therefore, it can be assumed that his blood has passed from the vena cava via the heart to the aorta. If it now be reckoned how many ounces of blood are extruded below a medium tight ligature during the space of twenty to thirty pulsations, an estimate can be formed of how much in the meantime is passing through the other arm, the legs, the two sides of the neck and all the other arteries and veins of the body. All these parts will be receiving blood which has passed through the lungs and the ventricles of the heart, which means that it must return through the veins, 'since so great a quantitie cannot be furnished from those things we eat, and that it is far greater than is convenient for the nutrition of the parts' (p. 83).

It is in cap. 13 that Harvey comes to the proof that the blood returns to the heart through the veins and to the evidence afforded by the valves. He attributes their discovery to Fabricius, but bows to Riolan's suggestion that it was Sylvius who first saw them. He describes them as 'looking upwards towards the roots' of the veins, in pairs, 'looking towards one another equally and duly touching one another, insomuch that they are apt to stick together at the extremities, and to be joynd', so that they completely prevent any backward flow. But, Harvey adds, neither the discoverer of these valves, nor anyone since, has rightly understood their use. They are not designed to prevent the blood falling downwards by its own weight, for in the jugular veins the valves face downwards, nor to prevent apoplexy, nor to halt the blood at the

divarications and prevent it from all going into the larger branches, nor
to retard the motion of the blood from the centre to the periphery.

> But the Portals were meerly made, lest the blood should move from the
> greater veins into the lesser and tear or swell them; and that it should
> not go from the centre of the body to the extremities, but rather from
> the extremities to the centre. Therefore by this motion the small Portals
> are easily shut, and hinder anything which is contrary to them; for they
> are so plac'd and ordain'd, that if any thing should not be sufficiently
> hindred in the passage by the hornes of the foremost, but should escape
> as it were through a chinck, the convexity or vault of the next might
> receive it, and so hinder it from passing any further (p. 86).

Harvey then describes his simple experiments with a probe which being
inserted into a vein in the direction towards the heart slid easily through,
but when inserted away from the heart encountered such resistance
from the valves that by no means could it be pushed beyond them. He
then proceeded to perform on an arm ligated for venesection the experiment that he had probably seen Fabricius do at Padua,[11] and at this
point he illustrates his book with its only picture, borrowed from
Fabricius's work on the valves of the veins, but with significant addi-
tional drawings. As the veins in this arm swell, the valves can be seen
as 'little nodes or swellings' and this is particularly obvious 'in country
people and those who are swoln vein'd'. If the blood be stroked away
from the heart towards the more distal valve, the portion of vein
between the two valves will remain empty. If you then with the other
hand try to push the blood back to fill the empty vein, you will find
it to be impossible. So the use of the valves of the veins may be compared
with the use of the sigmoid valves of the heart, namely to prevent the
regress of blood. Again, if you empty a portion of vein between two
valves and then remove the finger more distally placed, it will be
noticed that the vein refills immediately with blood moving towards
the heart. But all efforts to push the blood away from the heart back
through the valves will be found impossible. 'And do this a thousand
times'. And he adds a further reference to quantity:

> Now if you reckon the business, how much by one compression moves
> upwards by suppression of the portal, and multiplying that by thousands,
> you shall find so much blood pass'd by this means through a little part
> of a vein, that you will find yourself perfectly perswaded concerning the
> circulation of the blood, and of its swift motion (p. 90).

If you do not believe this, do it where the valves are far apart and you will find that the same phenomenon occurs.

With this Harvey has reached the end of all his experimental proofs of the circulation. Cap. 14 is brief, but contains a full and reasoned statement of the conclusion to which all these experiments and observations have inevitably led, the circulation of the blood.

> Seeing it is confirm'd by reasons and ocular experiments, that the blood does pass through the lungs and heart by the pulse of the ventricles, and is driven and sent into the whole body, and does creep into the veins and porosities of the flesh, and through them returns from the little veins into the greater, from the circumference to the centre, from whence it comes at last into the *vena cava*, and into the ear of the heart in so great abundance, with so great flux and reflux, from hence through the arteries thither, from thence through the veins hither back again, so that it cannot be furnished by those things which we do take in, and in a far greater abundance than is competent for nourishment: It must be of necessity concluded that the blood is driven into a round by a circular motion in creatures, and that it moves perpetually; and hence does arise the action and function of the heart, which by pulsation it performs; and lastly the motion and pulsation of the heart is the only cause (p. 91).

The remaining three chapters of *De motu cordis* are concerned with a diversity of subjects and observations, all of which follow once the circulation of the blood has been demonstrated and admitted, and they also contain some remarks on certain consequences in medical subjects which arise from it. When Harvey began to write, he obviously selected his material from a mass of accumulated observations and experiments, and this material he arranged according to a strictly rigorous plan. This precise selection and deliberate arrangement with a specific end in view is apparent in every chapter. The result is a work remarkable for the clarity of its exposition, but one which, perhaps, presents an over-simplification of the story. There are so many things left unsaid, so many difficulties undiscussed, because they are unnecessary for the establishment of the truth of the hypothesis. Because, in the central chapters of the book, Harvey argues at each stage from hypothesis through experimental proof of that hypothesis to conclusion, *De motu cordis* has just been justifiably acclaimed as the first work of 'modern' scientific writing. But at the same time, this praise obscures at least part of the merit of the book, for it takes no account of the difficulties in the way of this achievement. The notion of the circulation of the blood is now commonplace, and we know little and care less about the theories which its demonstration proved false, but unless some at least of these ideas are understood and their complexity and ramifications appreciated, Harvey's achievement is belittled. Only from this knowledge can we properly admire his capacity for bringing order out of chaos, the other facet of his ability for precise observation and clear and simple exposition. He began in what he himself calls a 'Labyrinth', and it is this which he discusses in the Introductory chapter.

Unlike the rest of *De motu cordis*, the Introductory chapter is designed to be destructive. It is an attack on what Harvey believed to be the major cause of prevalent error, the assumption that the beating of the heart and respiration fulfilled the same purpose and had the same use. The manifold errors, inconsistent notions and contradictory opinions arising from this belief, Harvey attacks and refutes. As the chapter proceeds it becomes clear that the experimental work which underlies it, is that which he probably first undertook to confirm the hypothesis of Columbus concerning the pulmonary transit of the blood.

> Almost all Anatomists, Physicians, and Philosophers to this day, do affirm with *Galen*, that the use of Pulsation is the same with that of Respiration, and that they differ only in one thing, that one flows from the Animal faculty, and the other from the Vital, being alike in all other things, either as touching their utility, or manner or motion (p. 1).

Even the most recently published work on the subject, Fabricius's *De respiratione*,[1][2] assumes that the lungs were made to fan and refrigerate the heart, because the pulse of the heart and arteries is insufficient for the purpose. So the systole and diastole of the heart had come to be related to the movement of the lungs, and that this supposition is pure nonsense, Harvey proceeds to make plain.

His first line of attack is to prove beyond all possible doubt that the arteries contain blood and not air. Starting from the premiss, if the arteries take in air in diastole and in systole expel fuliginous vapours, he refutes the conclusion that between these two movements they must contain air by citing Galen's work which proved it false. Not content with this, Harvey gives evidence from observation and experiment. It at once becomes clear that he is beginning at the very beginning of the subject, that he is not for the moment discussing respiration as we understand it, but the ancient notion which, for want of a better word, is usually called 'transpiration'. This notion underlies what Plato has to

136

say on the subject in the *Timaeus*, but its origin can be traced to Empedocles, who was the first to hold that the purpose of respiration was to control the natural heat of the body, and that respiration and the movement of the blood were one process. He believed that the air, together with the *pneuma* which was present in it, entered the body at the moment of inspiration not only through the mouth and nostrils, but also through the pores of the skin and the ends of the arteries underlying them. He thought that the alternate movements of inspiration and expiration were caused by the heart-beat. Thus, when the thin blood rushed back to the heart at the time of its diastole and left empty the extremities of the vessels lying under the skin, the air rushed in through the pores and was driven out again when the re-invigorated blood returned from the heart at the moment of expiration and systole. Later, it was thought that the air, and with it the spirit, went as far as the heart in its diastole, and from there, as being the centre of the 'breath-soul', $\psi\upsilon\chi\iota\kappa\acute{o}\nu$ $\pi\nu\epsilon\tilde{\upsilon}\mu\alpha$, of the body, was distributed to all the various parts along with the blood. At this date there was no clear distinction between veins and arteries. That came later, and with it the belief that the arteries, as their name implies, were empty of any content save air. Though Galen had conclusively proved in his attack on Erasistratus that the arteries did not contain air but blood, there were still among Harvey's contemporaries those who clung to the ancient opinion. Why they did so in the face of such patent evidence to the contrary is an unexplained marvel. It is this notion of transpiration which Harvey's first observations in this Introductory chapter refute. If a body is immersed in water or oil, the pulse neither falters nor changes as it should if the theory were true. Moreover, how can the foetus swimming in the womb, or whales or dolphins or all the fish of the sea take in air? 'To say that they sup up the air implanted in the water and do return their fumes into it is not unlike a fiction' (p. 3). (Maybe, in Harvey's time, but it is the truth nevertheless.) And if the air is given out this way, why not spirit as well? But Harvey is really attacking a notion that was already dead. I know of no anatomists in the century preceding Harvey who still believed in this doctrine in all its aspects. (Its vestiges remained for many years to come in folk-medicine: keeping the pores open, letting the body breathe through the pores of the skin.)

Experiments to prove that blood and not air is contained in the arteries follow. From a severed artery the blood is thrust out in a continual motion and air does not enter. When a limb is tightly ligatured, the parts beyond the ligature become cold; therefore the arterial pulse does not convey cooling air but warm blood. This experiment with the ligature is referred to in the Anatomical Lectures of 1616 (p. 269), and is the only one there mentioned. That blood and blood alone is contained in the arteries is proved by Galen's experiment in refutation of Erasistratus, by arteriotomy, and by the experience of wounds. Through the cut artery the whole body can be emptied of blood. These considerations all appear again in the main chapters of *De motu cordis*.

With regard to the arterial pulse, one remark is interesting because it probably relates to demonstrations that Harvey gave at the College of Physicians:

> But I believe I can easily demonstrate, and have heretofore demonstrated, that the arteries are distended because they are fill'd like Satchells or baggs, not because they are inflated like bellows (p. 6).

This observation and others which follow on the arterial pulse had all been made by 1616,[13] and Harvey uses them here to support his conclusion that the use of the pulse and the use of respiration are different and must not be confused simply because in certain conditions a like variation is found in both.

He then passes to problems more immediately connected with Columbus's discovery: the structure of the ventricles and of the valves of the heart, of the pulmonary artery and of the pulmonary vein. And in this connection he describes his experiment to prove that blood and not air is present in the pulmonary vein:

> If any would try the Experiment of *Galen*, and cut the wind-pipe of a dog being yet alive, and forcibly fill the lungs with air, and being filled bind them streight, afterwards cutting up his breast he shall find great store of air in the lungs, even to their utmost tunicle, but nothing in the *arteria venosa* [*sc.* pulmonary vein], nor in the left ventricle of the heart. But if in a living dog either the heart did attract it, or the lungs did pulse it through, they should do it much more in this experiment. Yea in the administration of Anatomy blowing up the lungs of a dead body, who doubts but the air would enter this way, if there were any passage? (p. 12)

After references to the foetal heart and the cardiac septum, Harvey comes to another point which he had already noticed in the Anatomical Lectures, the question of the voidance of pus from the chest through the urine. In the Lectures he had written: 'Into the renal vein is thrown a branch, sometimes two, from the azygos vein, hence matter from the chest is voided through the urine' (p. 169). In 1600, Andreas Laurentius in his *Historia anatomica* had questioned the truth of this view and reverted to the Galenic belief that pus from the chest is absorbed into the pulmonary vein, and thus goes to the left ventricle of the heart and into the arteries to the kidneys. The importance of this suggestion Harvey had not noticed in 1616. Here, in this Introductory chapter, he quotes Laurentius and concludes:

> But I cannot chuse but wonder, since he had guess'd and foretold that Heterogenous matter could be evacuated by the same passage, that he either could not or would not see or affirm, that through the same wayes the blood could be conveniently, according to Nature, brought out of the lungs into the left ventricle (p. 15).

It was the realisation of the incompatibility and impossibility of these many diverse notions concerning the movement of the heart and of the blood and of the lungs, that had led Harvey to the conclusion that much more work had to be done, not only on man but on animals, before a satisfactory answer could be given to the problem. And all this was completed before he began to write *De motu cordis*.

The last three chapters of the book form, as it were, a tail-piece to the whole, for they contain arguments *a posteriore*. They are concerned with topics relevant to the circulation and with phenomena that can be explained by it, once the hypothesis that the blood does circulate has been proved. Chapters 16 and 17 are chiefly concerned with matters medical and physiological and we will review them before turning to Harvey's more philosophical speculations concerning the circulation which are contained in cap. 15.

It is with the consideration of certain medical phenomena that Harvey begins cap. 16. The fact that the blood circulates through the body explains the generalising of infection consequent upon the bite of a venomous snake or a mad dog, and it also accounts for the symptoms of syphilis, the symptoms and post-mortem findings of tertain ague, explains the beneficial effects of medicaments externally applied and why a prognosis can be made from the pulse.

> Lastly, in all parts of Physick, Physiological, Pathological, Semeiotick, Therapeutick, when I do consider with my self how many questions may be determined, this truth and light being given; how many doubts may be solved, how many obscure things made clear, I find a most large

field, where I might run out so far and enlarge my self so much, that it would not only swell into a great volume, which is not my intention, but even my lifetime would be too short to make an end of it (pp. 100–01).

In this chapter also Harvey sketches the portal circulation and denies the two-way passage of blood and chyle in any vessel. It is to be noticed that he cites no experimental proof. The portal circulation followed by inference from the general and only later was he to devise its experimental proof. Here he passes on to the consideration of the part played by the liver in the adult and in the foetus and includes the observation, already made in 1616, that he had seen a foetus in which all the members were formed but the liver a shapeless mass of blood. Merely stating that the chick is formed and nourished in the egg from the white part only, and that the yolk serves it for nutrition after birth, Harvey leaves these questions of generation to pose, without answering, the problem of the order of the formation of the parts: why is the heart first formed? why does the blood exist before the heart? He concludes the chapter with an account of the contents of the splenic branch of the portal vein, an account totally different from that which he had given in 1616.[14]

Many of the observations which he had made before 1616 and which occur in the Lectures, Harvey repeats in cap. 17, which is obviously therefore based to a considerable extent on work done many years before the writing of De motu cordis was begun. Its chief topic is the heart and the manner of its action, and it reveals Harvey's remarkable knowledge of comparative anatomy and shows his manner of work applying these observations made on animals to the human body. It begins with remarks on the hearts of animals of many different kinds, on the foetal heart and on the relation of the heart and lungs. Then comes a discussion of the ventricles and of their strong fibrous bundles designed to assist contraction and wrongly called 'nerves' by Aristotle. Though Harvey does not here refer to Columbus by name, it is possible that he had his De re anatomica in mind, for Columbus had made the same point saying that Aristotle had been deceived into thinking them nerves and consequently into believing that the heart was the origin of sensation and movement.[15] Columbus himself believed them to be designed to strengthen and contain the valves of the heart. Harvey thought that it was the filaments of the mitral valves which possibly misled Aristotle into his belief in a three-chambered heart.[16] After a further discussion

140

of the action of the auricles, Harvey repeats the whole of his conclusions on the manner of the heart's action:

> It is likewise manifest that the ears do beat and contract themselves, as I said before, and cast the blood into the ventricle, whence it is that wheresoever there is a ventricle there an ear is requir'd, not only (as is commonly believed) that it may be the receptacle and cellar of blood (for what needs there any pulsation for the retaining of it?), but the first movers of the blood are the ears, especially the right, being the first thing that lives, and the last that dies, as before is said; for which cause they are necessary, that they may serve to pour the blood into the ventricle. But the ventricle immediately contracting itself, doth more conveniently squeeze out and more violently thrust forth the blood, being already in motion; as when you play ball, you can strike it further and more strongly, taking it *à la vole*, than you could only throwing it out of your hand. But likewise, contrary to vulgar opinion, because neither the heart, nor any thing else can so extend it self as that it can attract any thing in its diastole (unless in its return to its former constitution, being before squeezed like a spunge); but it is certain that all local motion comes first, and did take its beginning from the contraction of some particle; therefore by the contraction of the ears, the blood is cast into the ventricle as I open'd before, and by the contraction of the ventricle, it's thrown further and removed (pp. 110–11).

It is tempting to think that Harvey is here groping for the idea of the pacemaker, but in view of what he also says about the obscure ebullition in the blood it is clear that he had no real understanding of the cause of the heart's movement. What he did realise was that the heart is a muscle and that in its contraction it acts like a sphincter for its fibres are circular and not straight, transverse and oblique. When its fibres contract, they contract simultaneously, the apex is drawn to the base by the fibrous bundles, the walls come together concentrically, the whole heart contracts down everywhere and the ventricles are narrowed.

> Wherefore since the action of it is contraction, we must needs imagine that the function of it is to thrust blood out into the arteries (p. 114).

The final problems to be discussed in this chapter concern the differences between veins and arteries, and in particular the pulmonary vein and artery. All these phenomena and many more to be observed in dissections seem to have only one explanation, the circulation of the blood.

So far, there is little in *De motu cordis* on the purpose of the circulation. Harvey is too concerned to prove that his hypothesis is grounded on physiological and anatomical fact to waste time in this treatise on speculation. The subject is, however, glanced at briefly in cap. 8 and in cap. 15: 'The circulation of the blood is confirm'd by probable reasons.' It contains little, if anything, that is new. By means of statements from Aristotle, Harvey conducts the argument to the conclusion that the circulation is a logical necessity. Starting from Aristotle's proposition that death is cold and life is warm, and therefore, all living things are possessed of a source of innate heat from which warmth and life are dispensed or communicated to the parts, Harvey asks for it to be conceded with Aristotle that the heart is this source of innate heat and that, therefore, in this particular, the heart is to be considered as the *principium vitae*. He is, of course, not here thinking in terms of embryological development. He is not stating that in this sense the heart is the 'beginning' of life, but simply that, in those creatures which have hearts, the heart is the 'principal' of life, the source of the power to continue to live. In confirmation of this, Harvey points to the fact that the heart alone of all the parts of the body contains blood for the general use of the parts. The blood for its own use is conveyed to it by the coronary veins and arteries. Therefore, as Aristotle had said, the heart is to be considered as a storage cistern. The reasons for which Harvey dismissed the ancient Galenic belief that the liver fulfilled this rôle, he does not mention. They can be found in the Anatomical Lectures and again in *De generatione*,[17] but here in *De motu cordis* the discussion of the embryological findings on which his views were based have no place. Harvey is merely stating his conclusion, and it is a conclusion in which there is no novelty. If it be conceded that the blood, removed from the source of warmth, becomes cold and almost congeals, another Aristotelian maxim, the question to be answered falls into two parts: first, how to get the warm blood to the parts to ensure that they continue to live, and second, how to ensure that this blood does not get cold and 'die' at the periphery. The ancients had answered the question by the notion of perpetual ebb and flow. They were not clear how the blood got to the parts, whether by attraction or impulsion, or how it returned, or indeed how much of it returned, but they thought that the natural movement was always towards the centre from which it came, that is, towards the heart. So Harvey fits his new physiological facts into an Aristotelian framework and in the fitting there is no logical error or hiatus. The heart by its central position dispenses the blood 'as out of a treasure and fountain'.

Moreover to this distribution and motion of the blood, violence, and an impulsor is requir'd, such as the heart is. To this add, that the blood does easily concentricate and joyn of its own accord to its beginning, as a part to the whole, or as a drop of spilt water upon the table to the whole mass. . . . Besides, it is squeezed out of the hair-like veins into the little branches, and from thence into the greater, by the motion of the members and muscles: Likewise the blood is apter to move from the circumference to the centre than otherwise, though the portals did not hinder [*sc.* even if there were no valves to oppose its movement]. From whence it follows, that if it do leave its beginning, and move against its will, and enter into places narrower and colder, that it has need of violence and an impulser, such is the heart only, as we said but now (p. 95).

In one paragraph, Harvey steps outside his physiologically based speculations to subscribe in some measure to the ancient belief in the effect of the emotions on the heart. This does not mean that he is thinking of the heart as the seat of the emotions in the Aristotelian manner, but rather that strong emotions have a physical effect on the body and this physical effect is manifested in the behaviour of the heart.

And hence perchance the reason may be drawn, why in those that with grief, love, cares, and the like are possessed, a consumption or continuation happens, or cacochymie, or abundance of crudities, which cause all diseases and kill men. For every passion of the mind which troubles men's spirits, either with grief, joy, hope, or anxiety, and gets access to the heart, there makes it to change from its natural constitution, by distemperature, pulsation, and the rest, that infecting all the nourishment and weakening the strength, it ought not at all to seem wonderful if it afterwards beget divers sorts of incurable diseases in the members and in the body, seeing the whole body in that case is afflicted by the corruption of the nourishment, and defect of the native warmth (p. 94).

There seems to be little difference in this point of view from his belief that the circulation of the blood explains the generalising of infection consequent upon a poisoned wound and in certain diseases.

In spite of the fact that in *De motu cordis* Harvey stresses the central rôle of the heart, describing it in Aristotelian terms as the sun in the firmament, the dispenser of life, and so forth, it must be remembered that he holds this view only when speaking of the importance of the heart in the circulation of the blood, for at the same time he is fully aware that the heart does not hold this central rôle in the embryological development of the body. His investigations into the developing egg and mammalian ovary have already shown him that it is the blood and not the heart which first appears and consequently that it is the blood which is the primary source of life. To this he also refers in *De motu cordis*. This antithesis between the heart and the blood is fundamental to the whole of Harvey's writings and will be discussed later in connection with *De generatione*. Another topic, glanced at in *De motu cordis*, but which will also be more fitly discussed later in connection with *De generatione*, is that of the life which is inherent in the blood. It is linked with Harvey's views on the rôle of the blood and raises the whole question of his attitude to and belief in the existence of natural and vital spirits. These philosophical notions have no fundamental part to play in *De motu cordis* which remains pre-eminently the exposition and proof of a purely physiological hypothesis. It must not, however, be forgotten that they do underlie *De motu cordis* and that by divorcing them in this manner one is creating an artificial division in Harvey's thought. Their consideration is deferred merely for convenience in exposition. The proper understanding of *De motu cordis* can only be had from the knowledge of the whole of Harvey's thought.

NOTES

1. See above pp. 69, 94–5. See also p. 141 for Harvey's further discussion of the manner of the heart's action in *De motu cordis*, cap. 17, p. 114.

2. 'As we may see when a Horse drinks and swallows the water, at every gulp the water is sup'd down into the belly, which yields a certain noise and pulse to him that heeds him and touches him; even so it come to pass, that whilst some portion of the blood is drawn out of the veins into the arteries, there is a beating which is heard within the breast' (pp. 36–7). It was remarked by Kenneth D. Keele, *William Harvey*, 1965, p. 131, that this is the first mention to have been made by any anatomist of cardiac sound. He also alludes, p. 92, to the fact that Emilius Parisanus in 1647 made sarcastic comment on these noises, saying: 'Neither we poor deaf ones, nor any other doctor in Venice, can hear them, but happy is he who can hear them in London'.

3. Columbus had made similar points in his impassioned appeal for belief.

4. The use of the words 'the whole mass of the blood' is interesting in this context for it plainly relates to the pulmonary transit and to the pulmonary transit alone. Harvey has not yet announced the hypothesis of the circulation. It follows, therefore, that when he used these words in the Anatomical Lectures of 1616 (p. 297), this was the meaning he attached to them, and they must not be read as having any other connotation.

5. The translation is correct; the Latin has *attrahitur*.

6. This is the reverse of the opinion which Harvey expressed in the Anatomical Lectures where he says: 'the left ventricle is wanting and not, as is commonly supposed, the right' (p. 255). Presumably he was then thinking of the pulmonary transit of the blood only and changed his mind after formulating the hypothesis of the circulation.

7. Presumably intended for his projected work on Respiration. For a brief discussion of his views on this subject see my Introduction to *The Anatomical Lectures*, pp. liii–lvi.

8. See below p. 165.

9. See below p. 228.

10. Sanctorius (1561–1636) took his doctorate in medicine in Padua in 1587 and after fourteen years of service in Poland as physician to the King and then to the Prince of Hungary and Croatia, returned to practise in Venice from whence in 1611 he was called to be First Professor of the Theory of Medicine in Padua. He gave up the chair in 1624 and retired to his practice in Venice where he remained until his death. He was considerably influenced by the ideas of Galileo and modified devices invented by the astronomer for use as a thermometer, a clinical thermometer and a 'pulsilogium' or pulse meter. These and other instruments he describes in his commentary on part of the first book of the *Canon* of Avicenna printed in Venice in 1625. In his *De statica medicina*, Venice 1614, he describes a balance designed to measure the weight of the body at different times and demonstrates the fact that it loses weight by mere exposure, a process which he ascribed to 'insensible perspiration'. Though this book went through many editions and was translated into several languages, Harvey does not refer to it in any of his writings.

11. See above pp. 22–3.

12. Fabricius's treatise was published in 1615. Harvey describes it here as *nuperrime edito* which translators have taken to mean 'recently' or 'very recently published'. As Harvey cannot have been writing this chapter before 1619, it seems more likely that he is alluding to it as the 'most recently published' book on the subject. Otherwise the remark seems to have no particular relevance.

13. The statement that Galen's experiment with the pervious reed is impossible, that the systole of the heart coincides with the diastole of the arteries, and that the pulse of the arteries is not in their coats, as he proves by the instance of an aneurysm whose pulsation coincides with that of the artery although its coat is wanting.

14. 'The blood returning through those veins by both ways, and carrying the rawest juice with it, (hence from the ventricle, that which is waterish and thin, the chilifaction being not as yet perfected; from thence that which is gross and terrestial) in this branch of the splenick, by the permixtion of contraries, it is

conveniently temper'd; and Nature mixing those two juices of more difficult concoction, by reason of their contrary indispositions, with great abundance of warm blood, which (by reason of the abundance of arteries) flows abundantly from the milt [sc. spleen], it brings them, being now better prepar'd, to the *porta* of the liver, and supplies and recompences the defect of both by such a structure of the veins '(pp. 101–02).

15. 'In this great Aristotle was much deceived, for he thought that the filaments of which I am speaking were nerves and so it happened that Aristotle left it in writing that the heart was the origin of the nerves and, consequently of sensation and movement', *De re anatomica*, Bk VII, p. 179.

16. '. . . therefore in the left ventricle, that for the greater impulsion there may be a closer stoppage, there are only two like a Mitre, having tendons reaching out far, even to the *conus* of it, through its middle, that they may be most exactly shut. This perchance deceiv'd *Aristotle*, in making him believe that this ventricle was double, the division being made athwart, lest the blood should fall back again into the arterie . . .' (p. 109).

17. See below pp. 216ff, 221.

Controversy and Final Assessment

Chapter Seven

Reception and Controversy 1629–1648

FOR twenty years following the publication of *De motu cordis* controversy raged, as Harvey had expected, and during these years he
remained aloof from the debate. He published no reply to his critics
until 1649, when he at last answered the attacks of Jean Riolan the
younger of Paris with two letters, or *Exercitationes duae anatomicae de
circulatione sanguinis*. Little of his correspondence during this period has
survived, and only one of these surviving letters, that written to Caspar
Hofmann in 1636, is concerned with the circulation of the blood. It is
difficult to know what Harvey might have said to his critics beyond
re-affirming his theory, and of this there was no real need, given the
clarity and perfection of the exposition in *De motu cordis*. There was no
arguing with those who obstinately refused to believe a manifest truth.
His feelings are almost certainly revealed in a remark in *De generatione*,
which was being written during these years although it remained unpublished until 1651: 'I would say with Fabricius, "Let all reasoning be
silent when experience gainsays its conclusion". The too familiar vice
of the present age is to obtrude as manifest truths, mere fancies, born
of conjecture and superficial reasoning, altogether unsupported by the
testimony of sense.' Or again, speaking of an anatomical error made by
Fabricius because he had been misled by a popular notion: 'So it happens
to all who, forsaking the light which frequent dissections of bodies and
familiar converse with Nature supplies, expect that they are to understand from conjecture and arguments founded on probabilities, or the
authority of writers, the things or the facts which they ought themselves
to behold with their own eyes, to perceive with their proper senses.'
No one could advance against the circulation an argument worth a
moment's pause, no one could devise an experiment to demonstrate

149

its falsity. As Henry Power wrote in 1652 in his treatise *Circulatio sanguinis; inventio Harveiana*:[1]

> Amongst all the rabble of his antagonists, wee see not one that attempts to fight him at his own weapon, that is by sensible and anatomical evictions to confute that which he has by sense and autopsy so vigorously confirmed.

The first notice of Harvey's book to appear in print was favourable. It came from his friend Robert Fludd and appeared in the book *Medicina catholica* printed in Frankfurt in 1629. Fludd accepted the discovery because it fitted with his own philosophical ideas. Whether he had any real understanding of its physiological necessity is open to question in view of the fact that, in the following year, Pierre Gassendi, in a discussion of Fludd's whole philosophy, was of the opinion that Fludd accepted the circulation only in a mystical way, and added that he would have done better had he listened to Harvey.[2] But what Fludd made of the discovery was nothing to Harvey.

The first attack on *De motu cordis* came in March 1630 from James Primerose in a book, *Exercitationes et animadversiones in librum de motu cordis et circulatione sanguinis*, written expressly for that purpose and printed in London. As Primerose had been admitted a Licenciate of the College of Physicians only in the preceding December (when Harvey himself was one of the examiners), it seems likely that he was at that very time meditating this attack. In the book Primerose shows himself a convinced Galenist of the most conservative type and completely incapable of understanding Harvey's experimental evidence. He denies everything but refutes nothing. For instance, he deals with Harvey's Prefatory chapter in the following manner: it is not a new idea, to say that respiration and the pulse have different uses; Galen was of this opinion. The pulse does vary when a man is in the bath, as Galen said. Fish do not breathe in water. Pulsation is a 'virtue' of the heart, as Galen said. The coats of the arteries are not thicker to withstand the impulse of blood, but to keep in the spirits. There is a double movement in the pulmonary vein and it is similar to the movement of blood and chyle contrary ways in the portal vein, and the existence of this movement proves the existence of the former. And so on. There is not a single experiment in the whole book, nothing but quotations from authority, and chiefly from Galen and Vesalius. As Primerose had at one time been a pupil of Riolan, he naturally believes in the existence of pores in the septum of the heart. He explains away the fact that they cannot be found in dissection on the grounds that they fall together after death, but that 'when the heart beats and is contracted and dilated, then the pores in it in some manner also collapse and are dilated' (Ex. 25, p. 40). In any case these pores were seen, so he asserts, by Vesalius, Bauhin and Riolan. Only Columbus failed to see them, and, in consequence had to devise a most inconvenient route for the blood and one full of great difficulties. It is not surprising that Harvey refrained from replying.

Primerose was not alone in giving this explanation of the difficulty of finding the intraventricular pores. Thomas Winston in the Lectures which he delivered at Gresham College from 1615 onwards, and which were published posthumously in 1659, said of them that they 'cannot be seen in dead men for they fall together' (p. 179). And Winston had been associated with Harvey in the publication of the Pharmacopoeia produced by the College of Physicians and had served as Censor ten times between 1622 and 1637. It is to be believed that he must at least have known of Harvey's discovery, even if he did not assist at its demonstration.

In 1635, Emilius Parisanus joined in the attack on Harvey with a publication in Venice of Harvey's De motu cordis, interspersed paragraph by paragraph with what he supposed to be refutations of Harvey's proofs. To follow the controversy in detail through the next twenty years would be tedious and unprofitable. Not one of his opponents seems to have been able to suggest to Harvey any new train of thought, except Riolan, for whose benefit and the benefit of all convinced Galenists he gave new experimental proofs of the circulation, and not one of Harvey's supporters added anything to the subject.[3]

It was in 1632, and before he had seen a copy of De motu cordis, that Descartes arrived at the conclusion that the blood circulated throughout the whole body, and he set down his opinions in the treatise that he was then writing, the Tractatus de homine. This conclusion was based on a certain amount of dissection and observation, but was reached chiefly through ratiocination from basically Aristotelian and Galenic notions, and fitted into Descartes's concept of man as a machine. Briefly put, his theory was as follows. The blood leaving the liver is conveyed through the vena cava to the right ventricle of the heart which it enters drop by drop. As each drop encounters the heat of the heart, it is warmed, expands and becomes more subtle, in other words, is volatilised. At the moment of systole these exhalations of blood are driven into the pulmonary artery and so into the lungs. In the process they cool and condense again into blood. From the ends of the pulmonary artery, this blood enters the ends of the pulmonary vein and so returns to the left ventricle of the heart where a similar process occurs, the blood again entering only drop by drop. During the disatole of the heart, the valves of the veins of the heart open to allow one drop of blood from the vena cava and one from the pulmonary vein to enter each ventricle. As the blood is heated, it swells and closes the valve behind it to prevent any more from entering; but the expanding blood pushes open the valves of the arteries, and so, when the heart is in systole, the blood goes out through them. As the blood enters the aorta, it cools, and this arterial blood is carried into every part of the body. There by a process akin to digestion, some part of it is used up, but by far the greater part passes from the ends of the arteries into the ends of the veins and through the veins returns back to the heart, the valves in the veins preventing it from flowing in any other direction. 'So the movement of the blood in the body is nothing but a perpetual circulation.'[4]

> La plupart [sc. of the arterial blood] retournent dans les veines par les extrémités des artères, qui se trouvent en plusieurs endroits jointes à celles des veines. Et des veines il en passe peut-être aussi quelques parties en la nourriture de quelques membres : mais la plupart retournent dans le coeur, puis de là vont derechef dans les artères : en sorte que le mouvement du sang dans le corps n'est qu'une circulation perpétuelle (p. 811).

The position of the valves in the veins ensures the flow of blood towards the heart.

> Le sang qui est dans ses veines s'écoule toujours peu à peu de leurs extrémités vers le coeur (et la disposition de certaines petites portes, ou valvules, que les anatomistes ont remarquées en plusieurs endroits le long de nos veines, vous doit assez persuader qu'il arrive en nous tout le semblable) . . . (pp. 810–11).

If Descartes realised the use of the valves of the veins solely from their position and structure, one may well wonder why no anatomist before Harvey understood their meaning.

Though Descartes may have heard of Harvey's book from Mersenne some time during the winter of 1628–9 while he was on a visit to Paris, he did not see a copy of it until the autumn of 1632, after he had written the foregoing description, as is clear from the letter he then wrote to Mersenne:

J'ay veu le livre de Motu cordis dont vous m'aviez autresfois parlé, et me suis trouvé un peu different de son opinion, quoyque je ne l'aye veu qu'aprés avoir achevé d'ecrire de cette matiere.[5]

Having read the book and being convinced of the truth of the circulation of the blood, Descartes revealed his enthusiasm in a letter written to an unnamed correspondent, probably in England, some time between 1632 and 1637:

Ne connoissez vous point a Londres un médecin célèbre, nommé Hervaeus, qui a fait un livre de Motu cordis et circulatione sanguinis? Quel homme est-ce? Pour le mouvement du coeur, il ne dit rien qui ne fust desja en d'autres livres, et je ne l'approuve pas entierement. Mais pour la circulation du sang il y triomphe et a l'honneur de s'en estre avisé le premier, en quoy toute la medicine luy est fort redevable. Il promettoit quelques autres traittez; je ne sçay s'il a rien fait imprimer depuis. Car ce sont de tels ouvrages qui meritent d'estre vus, et non pas un grand nombre de gros volumes, qui ne servent qu'à employer ou barbouiller du papier.[6]

Thereafter Descartes never ceased to give Harvey credit and praise for his discovery. In the *Discours de la méthode*, published in 1637, he publicly proclaimed his belief in and acceptance of Harvey's hypothesis. Prior to that date he had performed a number of dissections and probably repeated some of Harvey's experiments. Before discussing the subject of the movement of the heart and arteries in the *Discours*, Descartes insists that those who know no anatomy should see at least one dissection in order to understand what he is about to say.[7] The description of the heart's movement which follows differs little from that already given in the *Tractatus de homine*, but is accommodated to Harvey's account in so far as the auricular and ventricular contractions are concerned. Of the circulation of the blood he wrote:

Mais si on demande comment le sang des veines ne s'épuise point, en coulant ainsi continuellement dans le coeur, et comment les artères n'en sont point trop remplies, puisque tout celui qui passe par le coeur s'y va rendre, je n'ai pas besoin d'y répondre autre chose que ce qui a déjà été écrit par un médecin d'Angleterre, auquel il faut donner la louange d'avoir rompu la glace en cet endroit, et d'être le premier qui a enseigné qu'il y a plusieurs petits passages aux extrémités des artères par où le sang qu'elles reçoivent du coeur entre dans les petites branches des veines, d'où il va se rendre derechef vers le coeur; en sorte que son cours n'est autre qu'une circulation perpétuelle (p. 160).

And Descartes states that this fact of the circulation is proved by the experiments with ligatures of varying tightness, by the valves of the veins and by the fact that all the blood in the body can be emptied through a severed artery.

But Descartes was never to agree with Harvey on the question of the heart's action. It would seem that Descartes derived his opinion of the movement of the heart from his own particular conception of the heat which was present in it. That he had taken this opinion from tradition is clear enough. He describes this heat variously, as a fire without flame, 'un de ces feux sans lumière', like heat generated in a hay-stack, or in fermenting wine in certain conditions, and so forth. He thinks that it is situated in the flesh of the heart, whose walls are consequently always sufficiently hot to cause any liquid touching them to evaporate. To explain this conception he uses the analogy of boiling milk which expands, thus showing that Aristotle's idea of ebullition in the heart had played some part in the evolution of his own opinion. He believes, also on the strength of ancient opinion, that the heart is the hottest member of the body, and moreover that the left ventricle is hotter than the right, and he thinks that this is proved because the left ventricle is larger than the right and the surrounding flesh thicker. (At this time many anatomists, influenced by their post-mortem findings of a larger cavity but a thinner wall, gave it out that the right was the larger of the two ventricles.) To explain the movement of the heart, he rejects the ancient belief that this was occasioned by its 'pulsific faculty', and substitutes in its place a purely mechanical explanation derived from his opinion concerning its heat. He seems to envisage the heart as a kind of motor driven by a series of explosions. Harvey's account did not make him change his mind, and in the *Discours* he explains how his view is to be preferred, firstly because it has a mathematical explanation, and secondly because it explains some of the phenomena unaccounted for in Harvey's thesis, notably the difference between venous and arterial blood.

> La différence qu'on remarque entre celui qui sort des veines et celui qui sort des artères ne peut procéder que de ce qu'étant rarefié et comme distillé en passant par le coeur, il est plus subtil et vif, et plus chaud incontinent après en être sorti, c'est à dire étant dans les artères, qu'il n'est un peu devant que d'y entrer, c'est à dire étant dans les veines (p. 161).

The other point on which Descartes disagreed with Harvey was over the systole and diastole of the heart, for he adopted the incorrect traditional view. In his *Description du corps humain*, published in 1648, he maintains that on this point Harvey is in error and that the cavities of the heart are not larger when it is elongated. Descartes even suggests an experiment to prove his thesis, though without realising that it could prove the contrary of what he supposes. If you cut off the tip of the heart of a living dog and put a finger into one of the ventricles, the blood will be felt pressing against the finger each time that the heart lengthens, whereas when it shortens, this pressure ceases. Moreover, if, as Harvey says, the heart becomes harder because the fibres constrict, then it must become smaller in size; but if it becomes harder because it is dilated by the inflowing blood, then it must increase in size. Calling observation to witness, Descartes concludes: 'Or, on voit par expérience qu'il ne perd rien de sa grosseur, mais qu'il l'augmente plutôt'.[8] That when the heart shortens and hardens its cavities become larger is to be proved also by another experiment. If you cut off the tip of the heart of a live rabbit, you can see that the ventricles are enlarged at the very moment that the heart hardens, and at this moment the ventricles drive out the blood. Even when only a few drops of blood are expelled because there is little blood left in the body, the ventricles still remain the same size. The fibrous bands in the ventricles prevent them from dilating any further under the pressure of the rarefied blood. According to Descartes's theory, therefore, the heart and its ventricles are enlarged at the moment that the blood is expelled.

The errors which Descartes has here made in his observations point very clearly to the extreme difficulty of watching a heart beat and analysing its movements. He seems to have thought that the heart was still in diastole when it was in fact passing into systole. What is difficult to understand is why he persisted in believing that the blood entered and left the heart only drop by drop, when, if he did perform the experiments he describes, he must have seen, as Harvey did, that the blood gushes out from the ventricle at each constriction. Perhaps, however, as he does not mention having cut an artery near the heart, he thought that the blood behaved differently in the intact animal. If he did not, then he did not control his theory by observation or experiment, a conclusion which the theory itself seems to warrant.

In his agreement with Harvey over the fact of the circulation of the blood and his disagreement over the heart's action, Descartes never varied. He joined in the quarrel in support of Harvey and waged battle with Plempius of Louvain whom he finally convinced. It was in a letter to Plempius, written in February 1638, that he carefully explained how his theory of the heart's action took into account the difference between arterial and venous blood, a fact which Harvey had overlooked in *De motu cordis*, and for which he was taken to task by many of his critics.

But for my own part I did not at all feare that objection, haveing explicated in [the *Discours de la méthode*] how this subitaneous rarefaction is made and what kind of ebullition the blood there suffers, for what can bee imagined capable to cause a greater and more suddaine change in the body, then this ferment I have described, and this boileing of the blood I spoake of. But perhaps you will say that the blood undergoes noe change when it leaves the arteries and goes into the veines, and soe the blood of the veines and arteries would not be different. For an exact answer to the difficultie, I desire you would first observe that there is not a dropp of blood in the Arteries that hath not passed a little before through the heart and that there allwayes remaines some dropps in the veines which have not passed through the Arteries (for it is knowne that allwayes some humour falls out of the Gutts into the veines), and soe all the veines with the liver ought to bee considered but as one vessell. This being put up, it is an easy thing to conceave that the blood ought to retaine the same qualities in the Arteries that it gott in the heart, for that if it were supposed it became white in passing through the heart, as it doth red in passing through the liver,[9] all the blood in the arteries would be white and that in the veines red, for the blood which incessantly should glide out of the Arteries into the veines, through never soe white, being mixed with the red blood of the veines, would presently become of its colour, just as water poured into wine takes the colour of wine. Moreover it is worth remarking that there are many things, that haveing beene heated, aquire qualities all together different from those they had by reason of their cooling suddainly or by degrees; for if you coole Glasse by degrees, it becomes soe fragile that it is not able to resist the force of aire, and wee see that the same thing is turned some time into iron, some time into steele according as it is differently tempered. Now one may compare the blood that is drawne out of an Arterie to a piece of glasse comeing red hote out of a furnace, and that which is drawne out of the veines to glasse heated by a slow fire. And even the fire of the most furious furnaces doeth not seeme to have so greate a force uppon steele or glasse as the moderate heate of the heart uppon the blood, a thing so susceptible of change, that it is corrupted by aire alone as soone as it hath left the veines.[10]

Though an interesting piece of reasoning from technological analogies, it unfortunately has little to do with what goes on in the body. Descartes is theorising and not looking.

The assertion by Harvey of the identity of venous with arterial blood was to prove a stumbling-block to several anatomists who had indeed observed the difference in colour between the two. One who raised this as an objection to Harvey's hypothesis was Johann Vesling, professor of anatomy at Padua. Although he had met Harvey in Germany earlier in the year, he wrote to him in December 1637 saying that, though he thought that the return of the blood to the heart through the veins was very likely, he did not understand the manner of it. In the various oviparous embryos that he had examined, he had found that 'in the arteries the blood is bright red, in the veins dark purple. The arteries move with an obvious systole, but expel nothing into the clear white liquid [sc. of the albumen]. The veins as usual lie quiet.' He asked Harvey to resolve his doubts. That Harvey did this is obvious from another letter which Vesling wrote subsequently to Fortunio Liceto, professor of philosophy at Padua, for in this he acknowledges his complete acceptance of Harvey's hypothesis. Unfortunately, Harvey's letter to Vesling is not now known to be extant. The same point was again raised in 1643 by Ole Worm of Copenhagen, who, since 1632, had been arguing against Harvey's theory. In 1643 he wrote to Thomas Bartholin saying:

> Have we not demonstrably shown that the blood in the arteries differs from that in the veins – differs in substance, colour, subtlety and all other properties? Bethink you, I pray, whether the blood in the arteries can possibly be that of the veins?[11]

Harvey's own views on the subject are to be found in the Second Letter to Riolan and will be discussed later.[12]

That Descartes devised his theory of the heart's action with a mechanical model in mind rather than from observation and experiment, he makes plain in a letter which he wrote on 5 July 1643 to the Dutch physician, Jan van Beverwijk. It is a reply to a request made by Beverwijk that he would tell him of 'the mechanical demonstrations by which, as I hear, you clearly establish the circulation of the blood.' Beverwijk had been a supporter of Harvey's views since at least 1637. Unfortunately, we do not know of his comments on the explanation which Descartes sent to him.

Although I am in complete agreement with Harvey concerning the circulation of the blood and look upon him as the first inventor of so great a discovery than which I think nothing greater or more useful in medicine, yet I entirely disagree with him over the movement of the heart. He would have it, if I remember aright, that the heart while it is dilating in diastole gives entrance to the blood into itself, and while it is contracting in systole voids it forth. I explain the whole process thus. When the heart is empty of blood, the new blood must needs enter into its right ventricle from the vena cava and into its left through the pulmonary vein; I say needs must because seeing that it is liquid and the orifices of those vessels which are wrinkled and form the auricles of the heart are wide open and the valves with which they are furnished opened, unless a miracle intervene, the blood must fall into the heart. Thereupon, after some blood has fallen into each ventricle, finding the heat there to be greater than in the veins out of which it fell, it perforce expands and needs more space than before; I say perforce, because such is the nature of blood, as is easy to prove by this, that when we get cold all the veins of our body contract and are scarcely to be seen, and afterwards when we grow warm again they swell so that the blood contained in them is seen to occupy ten times more space than before. When, therefore, the blood expands thus in the heart, suddenly and violently it pushes against the walls of the ventricles on all sides, with the result that the valves which are in the mouths of the vena cava and pulmonary vein are closed and those which are in the mouths of the pulmonary artery and aorta are opened, for such is the structure of these valves that, according to the laws of mechanics, the latter must be opened by the sole force of the blood and the former closed. And this expanding blood makes the diastole of the heart. But this same blood, by the self-same movement by which, being itself expanded in the heart, it opens the valves of the pulmonary artery and aorta, likewise drives before it all the other blood contained in the arteries, by which is made their diastole. Afterwards, that same blood with the same violent movement with which it is expanded, enters the arteries, and thus the heart is left empty, and in this its systole consists. And the blood which has been expanded in the heart when it reaches the arteries, is again condensed, because there the heat is not so great, and in this consists the systole of the arteries which in time differs little from the systole of the heart. But at the end of this systole, the blood contained in the arteries slides backwards to the heart, but does not enter the ventricles because such is the construction of the valves existing in their mouths that they are of necessity closed by this falling back of the blood. On the other hand, the valves which are in the mouths of the veins open of their own accord as the heart subsides, and so new blood glides from the veins into the heart and a new diastole begins. Now all these things are truly mechanical, as also the experiments are experiments in Mechanics by which it is proved that there are diverse anastomoses of veins and arteries through which the blood flows from the latter into the former, for instance concerning the position of the valves in the veins, the ligature of the arm for venesection, the issuing forth of all the blood in the body through a single vein or artery that is opened, etc. No futher things worthy of recounting occur to me in this matter. It seems to me so plain and so certain that to prove it with further arguments appears superfluous.[13]

Though such a system with a hot-chamber and a series of valves and pipes could perhaps be made to drive a fluid around in a circle, it would not have the least resemblance to the action of the heart.

In 1644, the cudgels were taken up on Harvey's behalf by his friend Sir Kenelm Digby, who in his book, *Two treatises*, published in Paris in that year, answered the views expressed by Descartes. First he denied that the movement of the heart was to be explained by the action of heat within it. Next, he denied that the heart was like 'limber leather' which is blown up and shrinks down like a bladder, having no motion of its own.

> Doctor Haruey prooueth that when it is full, it compresseth it selfe by a quicke and strong motion, to expell that which is in it: and that when it is empty, it returneth to its naturall dilatation, figure and situation, by the ceasing of that agents working, which caused its motion. Whereby it appeareth to be of such a fibrous substance, as hath a proper motion of its owne (p. 233).

Though he takes Descartes's ideas one by one and refutes each in turn, he effectively disposes of the whole argument by his reference to the fact that a viper's heart taken out and laid on a plate will beat for twenty-four hours and more. Descartes's theory requires the continual access of fresh blood to initiate the continued beating of the heart. The excised viper's heart is necessarily deprived of fresh venous blood, yet it beats 'without succession of bloud to cause the pulses of it'.

Because Descartes said that he deduced the circulation of the blood from the position and structure of the valves in the veins, and because they first 'hinted' to Harvey the possibility of the circulation, it is interesting to notice that Hermann Conring was one of the first to realise the important part they played in the evolution of the hypothesis. In his treatise *De sanguinis generatione et motu naturali*, printed in Leyden and Amsterdam in 1646, he says that the whole argument begins from these valves because they prevent the reflux of blood. After quoting Harvey's experiment of trying to press the blood downwards through the veins and finding its flow impeded in a living subject by a valve, Conring adds that in a dissection not even air can get past the valve if you blow towards the smaller veins. This was the same Conring who, in 1631, as a young student, had damped the eager enthusiasm of Jacob Schwabe for the new theory by saying: 'Certainly this explanation in itself is elegant, and, at first glance, highly probable. If Harvey had only been able to prove it by means of autopsies and anatomical demonstrations, he would have solved the problem.'[14] In the intervening ten years, Conring had confirmed the truth of Harvey's statements to his own satisfaction by experiments on dogs.

Some of the objections raised by the staunch followers of Galenic tradition and Harvey's replies to them are to be found in the letters exchanged between him and Caspar Hofmann in 1636. From 11 to 22 May 1636, Harvey was in Nuremberg, in the train of the Earl of Arundel, and the story of how on that occasion he met Caspar Hofmann, professor of medicine in the near-by university of Altdorf, and demonstrated to him the circulation of the blood is well-known. Hofmann had himself been educated in the medical school of Padua. He had been trained by Fabricius and had learnt of the existence of the valves of the veins, but he had not progressed to an understanding of their implication. He had, however, advanced beyond Fabricius's own views on the movement of the blood, for he denied the existence of pores in the septum of the heart and held instead that the blood passed from the right ventricle to the left by way of the lungs. Hofmann was one of the few anatomists of the period to be influenced by the work of Caesalpinus. He quotes his writings with admiration on various occasions when deviating from the traditional Galenic views. As a result, he bases his belief in the existence of the pulmonary transit of the blood on the dual function of the pulmonary artery: to convey the blood from the right to the left ventricle through the lungs, thereby ensuring its refrigeration; to supply the lung with necessary aliment. This transference of the blood he calls a 'circulation', using the word in the same sense as Caesalpinus, that is to say with the meaning attached to it by the alchemists,[15] and referring not to the movement of the blood in the vessels but to the action of cooling the hot blood. Although he ascribes the discovery of the pulmonary transit to Columbus,[16] he does not properly understand the significance of Columbus's work for he does not realise, as Columbus did, that this movement of blood through the lungs is a physiological phenomenon which follows as an immediate and necessary consequence from the competence of the valves of the heart. The size and the substance of the pulmonary artery merely support the idea of a large flow of blood through the lungs, and do not, as he supposes, prove it. Apart from this and a few other variations where he follows Caesalpinus and Aristotelian opinion, Hofmann's views on the blood and its movement were basically Galenic. He held with Caesalpinus that the heart (not the liver, as Galen taught) was the source of all the blood in the body, both arterial and venous, and believed this to be proved by the existence of numerous anastomoses between veins and arteries.[17] He thought that the heart concocted the blood to make it perfect nutriment for the parts which attracted and retained it through their own faculties. He did not understand the manner of action of the heart for he denied it to be a muscle: 'Imo totum hoc apud me est γελοῖον'.[18] Instead he attributed its movement to the action of the nerves.

It was in fulfilment of a promise given on the preceding day that, on 19 May 1636, Hofmann wrote a letter to Harvey giving his opinion on the circulation of the blood.

> My hope is that you will receive it in the spirit in which I send it to you, that is, without any trace of ill-will with which I might vex you, nor with any high-flown arrogance whereby I might seem to know more than you, but simply and sincerely. For which reason I give you my solemn promise that if, having dispelled the clouds, you will show me the TRUTH more beautiful than the morning and the evening star, I will with Stesichorus, make public recantation and withdraw from the field.

Part of the text of this letter was printed in a volume of letters, *Epistolae selectiores*, collected by G. Richter and published from Nuremberg in 1662. That it is only part is obvious from Harvey's reply to it written on the following day.[19] The complete text of Hofmann's letter is not now known to exist, but the greater part of it can be read in his *Digressio in circulationem sanguinis, nuper in Anglia natam*, which was included by Jean Riolan in his *Responsio ad duas exercitationes anatomicas postremas G. Harvei de circulatione sanguinis*, published from Paris in 1652. The

Digressio seems to be part of a manuscript on physiology (it is called 'Caput 48 Manuscripti Physiologici') which Guy Patin acquired from Hofmann and gave to Riolan. Though not identical with the original letter, the *Digressio* appears to incorporate verbatim the greater part of its contents. It contains every point which Harvey answers in his reply.[20]

Hofmann's criticism of the circulation rests on two objections. First, if it happens, why and for what purpose is it? Second, how does the blood pass from the arteries into the veins? The first is perhaps the greater difficulty for him; he can see no purpose in the circulation. He totally ignores Harvey's experimental proofs as set out in *De motu cordis* and limits himself to an attack on the various passages of ratiocination in the book. He begins by questioning the validity of Harvey's statement, contained in cap. 14, that more blood is driven from the heart into the arteries than can either be replaced by the ingested food or consumed by the parts.

> A few words, but weighty! But how will you prove it, my dear Harvey? For you would seem to accuse Nature of stupidity in that she went so far astray in a work of almost prime importance as is the making and distributing of food. . . . You would seem to impose upon Nature the character of a most rude and idle artificer who destroys the work she has done and perfected so that, forsooth, she should not be at a loss for something to do, for, to make raw again the blood that has been perfected by all her agents and then again to concoct it, what is it other than this?

As it was at this time the generally accepted assumption that the heart perfected the blood and distributed perfected venous blood through the veins and perfected arterial blood through the arteries to all the parts of the body, this objection raised by Hofmann is valid, if the assumption is valid. If, as Harvey maintained, this blood circulated through the body, then it was perforce subjected to an infinite repetition of the same process. It is not, therefore, surprising that Hofmann taunts Harvey with, on the one hand, expressly upholding the Aristotelian maxim that 'Nature is neither deficient in those things which are necessary nor redundant in those which are superfluous', while on the other making her engage in apparently unnecessary work.

Hofmann next accuses Harvey of abandoning anatomy for logistic and proceeds to the arguments from the quantity of blood expelled from the heart at each beat:

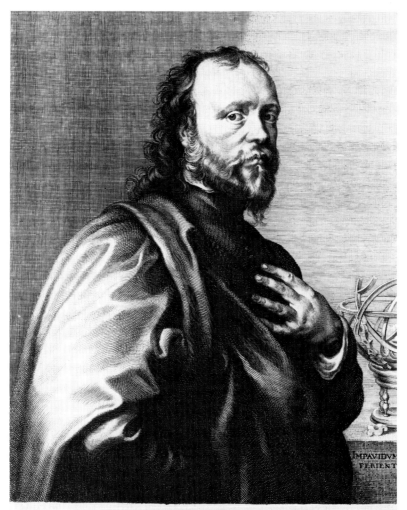

D. KENELMVS   DIGBI EQVES

R.V. Vorst sculp   Ant. van Dyck pinxit   Mart. vanden Enden excudit Cum priuilegio

V Sir Kenelm Digby

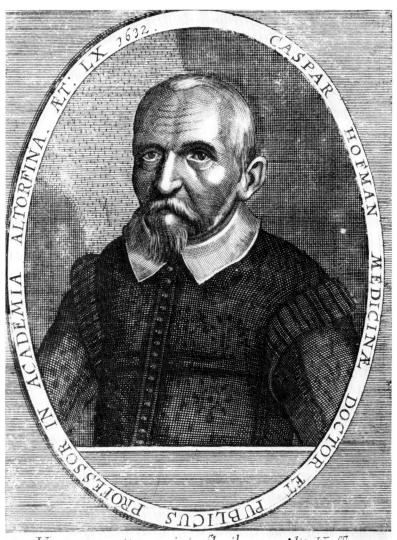

CASPAR HOFMAN MEDICINÆ DOCTOR ET PUBLICUS PROFESSOR IN ACADEMIA ALTORFINA. ÆT: LX 1632.

Hortorum vitas qui in floribus excòlit, Hoffman
Dicitur, et Medici quid magis ornat opus?

114.

VI *Caspar Hofmann in* 1632

Of a truth, you do not use your eyes or command them to be used, but instead rely on reasoning and calculation, reckoning at carefully selected moments how many pounds of blood, how many ounces, how many drachms have to be transferred from the heart into the arteries in the space of one half hour. Truly, Harvey, you are pursuing the incalculable, the inexplicable, the unknowable.

Because Hofmann believes in the ebullition of the blood, he is convinced that Harvey's reasoning is at fault and that he cannot possibly know the amount of blood passing through the arteries in any given time. Moreover, Primerose had also tried to make the calculation and he had concluded that it was not a matter of ounces and drachms, but of grains.

Primerose ... denies that there is much blood, nay more, he clearly asserts that there is but little, but it appears much on account of its swelling up, or, as I would say, its ebullition. Taking up the logistic of his adversary [i.e. Harvey], he comes from ounces and drachms to grains.

So Hofmann is not to be persuaded that the amount of blood is in excess of what can be produced by the food and consumed by the parts of the body.

And for what purpose is all this for which there is no foundation? where indeed, the phenomenon, το "οτι,[21] is not agreed, where it is hidden in the deep well of Nature, where the clearest reasoning is against it. . . . Eternally to no purpose.

Next, he denies that the movement of the bood in the veins is like that of water in a river in which, in some manner, one wave follows hard upon another and always flows downwards until it reaches the sea into which it empties itself. Instead, he asserts that it should be compared with the movement of the water in the sea itself, or in some stagnant pool where the wind sets the flow of the water in motion.

In this pool it is very likely that some of the water is always being absorbed into the bank, though no one could possibly measure the amount.

In support of this view he cites the opinion of Hippocrates in *De corde* concerning the 'surging', ζάλη, of the arterial chyle, and equates it with the pulsating of the blood in the arteries.

Hofmann now comes to the second part of Harvey's hypothesis that more blood than the parts need gets into the arteries. Here, he merely supports the views of Primerose to the effect that 'this is contrary to the wisdom of Nature who through the attractive faculty does not attract more than is necessary.' Though this is a Galenic principle, it overlooks the fact that it is impossible to tell how much is necessary. From this he passes on to the comment that if the parts did get more than the 'necessary' amount of blood they would be afflicted with perpetual inflammation, and questions Harvey's hypothesis that it is to prevent this from happening that the blood must return from the parts to the heart through the veins.

> Here I would like to learn from Harvey by what paths it goes out of the arteries into the veins? You do not say through their ends, for indeed they do not meet, nay they end in the flesh and form pores through which go the excrements of the third concoction and sometimes sweat. He says that it happens either indirectly through porosities in the flesh, or directly through an anastomosis. May I confess my bewilderment, I understand neither. Not indirectly through the porosities, because the blood which escapes from its vessels, and by this very act nourishes the part, does not return, nor can it return. Not directly, because in the parts to be nourished nobody ever dreamt of the existence of anastomoses. But they do exist in the greater vessels, although Harvey denies it in plain words. But let it be granted that invisible passages exist, unknown to so many preceding centuries and first seen by this Englishman, by what faculty is the backward movement made? The man replies, by the heart. Now the heart I know, according to Galen, *De usu partium*, Bk VI, cap. 15, attracts by all possible means, but how far does its power extend? to the parts that have to be nourished? I ask you. This is indeed a new and unheard of thing.

He believes that the pulse can drive the blood out from the heart but cannot possibly recall it to the heart because the attractive and retentive faculties of the parts themselves (a Galenic notion) prevent it. And he concludes:

> But let it be so to your good pleasure, as some say, to what purpose is it done? To be concocted a second time. To be concocted? Does it not, therefore, become raw again? Unless this happens, how is it that bile is not created rather than blood? For all physicians are of the opinion that in its final elaboration, blood is turned to bile, now yellow, now black. But let it be as you say, does not Nature concoct in order to concoct? And then afterwards concocts a second time? and repeats the process again a third time, and a fourth and so on for ever? To what purpose? I ask again.

On the following day, 20 May, Harvey wrote his reply. It is a little masterpiece of patient argument. Convinced of the validity of his experimental proofs he is certain that the phenomenon exists, but for what purpose he will not say, nor will he be easily made to hazard as much as a guess. He does not know precisely how the transference of the blood from the arteries to the veins does take place, but he is positive that it does occur, because it is a necessary event in the circulation of the blood which, for other reasons, must perforce go on in the body. There is no doubt that Hofmann's letter, typical as it is of the objections which could be raised by an orthodox Galenist, affords us some idea of the difficulties which Harvey encountered during these years.

Harvey begins his letter by denying the charge that he imputes to Nature the character of an idle artificer who destroys what she has perfected in order to remake it and so have something to do.

> But truly, since I do not know where or when such things were either said or thought by me who have always deemed myself an admirer of Nature's skill, wisdom and industry, it grieves me not a little to be taken for such a person by so fair-minded a man as yourself. In the little book I published, I merely assert that the movement of the blood from the heart through the arteries into the whole body, and likewise from the body through the veins back to the heart, is carried on continuously and without interruption, with such an outflowing and such an inflowing, with such quantity and abundance that it must of necessity move in some manner in a circle.

He denies that he has ever made any statement on the purpose of the circulation:

> But about concoction and about the causes of this movement and circulation, particularly about its final cause, I have never spoken, but have omitted it altogether, deliberately, and this you will find expressly stated if it please you to read again caps. 8 and 9. Indeed, you proceed to complain that I am a poor Anatomist and a poor Analytical Philosopher, simply because I try to investigate the phenomenon itself ($\tau\tilde{\phi}$ $"o\tau\iota$) without having established the wherefore ($\delta\iota\acute{o}\tau\iota$). I will love you sincerely and most affectionately if you will read the summary of all my assertions in cap. 14. You will discover that I add to the phenomenon ($\tauo\tilde{v}$ $"o\tau\iota$) nothing but the general account of it, that I add to it no physiological speculation, that I add no causes over and above, nor speculate for what reason Nature gives this motion to the blood by means of the beating of the Heart. I do not deny that in cap. 8 I insert in passing for the sake

of an illustration, as very likely may happen, that the parts may be warmed by means of the heat of the blood inflowing from the heart, and contrariwise that the blood may be weakened or suffer some accident in the parts, so that once again it returns to the heart and the fountain of heat for the sake of regaining its perfection. But whether this be so or not, I openly declare that I have not yet proved, or even said much about. Likewise, in the last chapters, I infer from my anatomical observations and their consequences that a circulation probably occurs, but nowhere do I set out its causes (save for the heart moving with its own pulsatory power).

Harvey now repeats that he has seen the circulation in many vivisections and shown it to a number of people. The arguments from the quantity of blood extruded at each heart beat confirm the circulation, no matter how imprecise a calculation is made of the quantity. If Hofmann would only look for himself he would see as clearly as he was shown in the demonstration that Harvey did for him on the preceding day, that the blood is diffused through the arteries into the whole body and that the blood from the smaller veins goes into the larger from every part of the body and so on up to the heart 'with as free a passage and confluence as your Pegnitz flows into the Regnitz, or the Regnitz into the Main, as the Main and the Mosel into the bed of the Rhine.' In fact, the arguments which Hofmann has so far advanced amount to nothing more than a statement that Harvey is a bad anatomist and a bad philosopher, and therefore, the circulation of the blood does not exist. 'But this is a non-sequitur.' Turning his attention to Hofmann's own analogy and comparison of the movement of the blood with the sea and with water in stagnant pools where the banks absorb moisture, Harvey politely holds it up to ridicule and turns the tables on Hofmann:

> Truly, my most learned and very dear friend, it would please me if you were now to smart for it. Surely, stagnant water does not flow? forgive me, I do not understand. Or as the water in the sea is in flux? The alternative proposition excites suspicion. But supposing it were as in the sea! There, there is such an inflowing and an outflowing at set times, and therefore the blood must go forwards and backwards in its vessels, and Nature would prefer the blood to be properly divided off and limited in the vessels rather than unlimited and disordered.[22] Moreover, why do the lands of Egypt not take in as much moisture from the Nile as it flows past as they would if it formed a pool of stagnant water! I do not understand.

Finally Harvey comes to answer the problem of how the blood passes from the arteries to the veins, and it is not so much an answer as an attack.

> The remainder of the points set out in your letter against the circulation are doubts of your own making because you refuse to accept porosities and invisible meanderings through the flesh. Without beating about the bush, you set up as obstacles to the contrary movements of expulsion and retention, the manner of the transit and the ways and faculties which you yourself postulate, and you ask for the final cause. . . . You say that the heart draws from the liver, why do the attractive and retentive faculties of the liver present no obstacle? and how does the blood come from the mesenteric veins to the vena cava, by what routes and vents, by means of an anastomosis, or in the very midst by means of the parenchyma of the liver? You never saw it, but you have no doubt that it may be. You do not hesitate to accept that the food is brought into the liver from the intestines through the tiny and hair-like ramifications of the portal vein, and at the same time that the blood is distributed into the intestines without any impediment, thereby affirming a contrariety of movement and a disorderliness.

All the objections which Hofmann has raised have already got their answers in *De motu cordis*, 'and they do not refute me'. Because the purpose of the circulation is unknown it does not follow that the phenomenon does not exist.

> He who would admit the circulation either by means of actual dissection or by an argument from probability, is not to be despised even though he may not know its ways or faculties, for such an investigation comes later, and from these matters arise too much contradiction and elenchic argument.

And at this point, Harvey gives up:

> Now I fear that truly you deem me too little of an Analytical Philosopher, assigning as I am causes and resolving doubts for him who perhaps will not admit that the phenomenon may be; for this is indeed the sophistical method and, as it were, to speculate about non-being.

If at any time Hofmann wants to see for himself the things which Harvey has said about the circulation, then, if the occasion serves, Harvey will come and demonstrate them to him.

> But if you neither want this nor will be pleased to search into the matter by your own efforts in dissections, please do not, I beg you, disparage

the work of others or ascribe it to error, or dishonour the word of an honest man who is not altogether unskilled nor a madman, in a matter which he has tested so many times over so many years.

As is well known, Hofmann was never to be persuaded of the truth of the circulation of the blood.

Harvey's letter to Hofmann does not show any development in his thought since the publication of *De motu cordis*. What is interesting about it is the way in which he never really meets the arguments of Hofmann. These arguments are not based on anatomical fact but on assumptions which cannot be demonstrated to be true or false, and are consequently exceedingly difficult to refute. If the heart does make the blood perfect, then unless it somehow loses this perfection before it returns to the heart, then the heart is re-perfecting the blood again and again. Harvey himself was not sure whether the heart did add anything or not beyond the motive force required. At one time he thought it added heat and consequently the blood which had cooled at the periphery returned for the purpose of regaining this heat. This he explains to Hofmann was merely a tentative suggestion. He was not sure whether the heat derived from the heart or from the blood itself. While he is himself perplexed about the purpose of the circulation, he can give no answer to Hofmann. He is fully aware that he does not know, and moreover, that any speculation which he may make is incapable of demonstration in an autopsy or a vivisection, and so incapable of proof. Again, with regard to the question of how the blood goes from the ends of the arteries into the ends of the veins, Harvey is also in a difficult position. He cannot see the capillaries, he cannot demonstrate the passage. He is well aware that he has denied the existence of anastomoses between veins and arteries. (His proof that they do not exist was to be published twelve years later in his Letter to Riolan.) He has also denied the existence of invisible pores in the septum of the heart. Yet here he must postulate the existence of something analogous in order to connect the arteries with the veins. He falls back on the analogy of the parenchyma of the liver, and instead of answering Hofmann, attacks him. He knew that Hofmann had too great a faith in the opinions of authority to believe the testimony of his own eyes. Consequently all Hofmann's arguments are frivolous and not one, except the argument from quantity, has anything to do with Harvey's exposition in *De motu cordis*.

★   ★   ★

It seems likely that it was during these years that Harvey saw the analogy which could be drawn between the action of the heart and that of a pump. The analogy does not occur in *De motu cordis* and it is unlikely that it formed any part of the original theory. Harvey's hypothesis was entirely formulated from anatomical and physiological evidence. Unlike that of Descartes, it was not developed with reference to any mechanical system and Harvey's use of the analogy to describe the action of the heart is largely a visual one. It occurs in his writings for the first time in the passage added subsequently on a blank page in the manuscript containing his notes for his Lectures on the Whole of Anatomy. The passage, as is well known, is a summary statement of the circulation, and its presence in this manuscript has been responsible in the past for leading many into the erroneous belief that when Harvey delivered these lectures for the first time in 1616, he was already aware of the existence of the circulation of the blood.

> WH it is certain from the structure of the heart that the blood is perpetually carried across through the lungs into the aorta as by two clacks of a water bellows to raise water. It is certain from the experiment of the ligature that there is a passage of the blood from the arteries to the veins. And for this reason $\varDelta$ it is certain that the perpetual movement of the blood in a circle is caused by the heart beat (p. 273).

The reference to the experiment with the ligature leads straight to *De motu cordis* but could have been added to the notes either shortly before the publication of that book or at any time later. It is the 'two clacks of the water bellows to raise water' that is of interest. A 'clack' is a valve and according to John Bate in his book *The Mysteries of Nature and Art*, published in London in 1634, it is 'a peece of Leather nayled over any hole having a peece of lead to make it lie close, so that the ayre or water in any vessell may thereby bee kept from going out' (p. 8). It had been thought for some time in the past that Harvey was referring to one of the many kinds of pumps used for drainage, but in a recent article Mr C. Webster has suggested that the pump which he had in mind was a fire-engine.[23] With this suggestion various pieces of evidence seem to fit. It was during the seventeenth century that water-mains were installed in the streets of many towns in England. They were made of hollowed logs of elm, the tapered end of one being fitted into the untapered end of the next, and the firefighters had merely to cut into the logs to allow the water to run into the street whence they scooped it up in leathern buckets. During the first quarter of the century also, fire-engines began to be used, but they were primitive and crude affairs. However, John Bate does describe two engines, both of which make use of a bellows pump and of 'clacks'. One of these is 'an Engin which being placed in water will cast the same with violence on high' (p. 11), the other an engine 'to force water up to a high place: very usefull for to quench fire amongst buildings' (p. 18). Though Harvey could be referring to one or other of these, the evidence is not conclusive. His next use of the analogy, however, in the Second Letter to Riolan, sheds more light on what he has in mind. He is describing the manner in which the blood spurts out from a cut artery at every contraction of the heart and says:

> Just as water, by the force and impulsion of a *sipho* is driven aloft through pipes of lead, we may observe and distinguish all the forcings of the Engine, even though it be a good way off, in the flux of the water when it passes out, the order, beginning, increase, end, and vehemency of every stroke (pp. 183–4).

Though the various translators have had different opinions as to the meaning of the word *sipho*, it is commonly used at this date for a fire-engine and the assumption that Harvey is describing such an engine fits well enough with what he says of it. It remains to discover why this visual analogy occurred to him and when.

The first description of a fire-pump of a kind that might have suggested it to him was published in 1615 by Salomon de Caus. He was an engineer in the service of Henry, Prince of Wales, and designed the fountains and waterworks for Henry's palace at Richmond; but he is chiefly remembered for the elaborate water-machines with which he ornamented the gardens of the Elector Palatine and his English wife, the Princess Elizabeth, in their castle at Heidelberg. In his book, *Les raisons des forces mouvantes*, he describes in Bk I, problem 20, an engine to be used to save burning houses. He says that this machine has been much used in Germany and can be of service even if the flames are forty feet high, for 'the said engine shall there cast its water by the help of four or five men lifting up and putting down a long handle in the form of a lever where the handle of the pump is fastened. The said pump is easily understood: there are two valves within it, one below to open when the handle is lifted up and to shut when it is down, and another to open to let out the water; and at the end of the said machine there is a man who holds the copper pipe, turning it from side to side to the place where the fire shall be.' As Salomon de Caus and Harvey both frequented the Court circle, it is not impossible for the two men to have known each other and for Harvey to have learnt of the pump either directly from de Caus or from his book. But the suggestion is an unlikely one, and it seems more probable that it was the sight of such an engine at work that supplied Harvey with the analogy. Though common in Germany, engines after this kind were not in use in London until about 1625 and even then they were rare. In 1637 a fire broke out near Arundel House in the Strand and one of these engines was used on that occasion with great success as is clear from a letter written by Charles I to the Lord Mayor of London ordering more to be provided:

> Whereas wee have had good information of the excellent use to be made in accidents of fire of the new Engine for spowting of water, and in the late fire which happened near Arundel House the good use thereof did manifestly appear, although there was none of the said Engines brought until it was late, by reason (as is informed) that there was none of the said Engines in the Parishes thereaboutes, We have thought fit to take notice to your Lordship of the great scarcity of the said Engines, considering the great use to be made of them, and earnestly to recommend unto you that there may a frequent provision be made of them, so as that upon all occasions, they may be near and ready to hand.[24]

Harvey had just returned to London after his journey across Europe with the Earl of Arundel. That he heard about the fire and perhaps even saw it is not impossible. The 'new Engine' obviously made a stir in London. It is, therefore, suggested that it was upon this occasion that Harvey saw the analogy with the fire-pump. Why, at so late a date as this, he should have added the summary statement of the circulation to his notes for the Anatomical Lectures remains unexplained.

Confirmation that it was the new fire-engine that suggested the analogy comes from the Anatomical Lectures of Francis Glisson delivered before the College of Physicians in London in 1653. There Glisson, speaking of the action of the heart, writes:

> This spouting out of the blood from the harte may be compared to the casting out of water by the engine of late invention for the quenching of

fire; as also to the squirting out of liquors by a syringe.[25] For if we cutt an artery we shall see the blood at every contraction of the harte to be darted out to a great distance, which showes the force of this contraction of the harte.[26]

It would be wrong to suppose that all the physicians and anatomists of Harvey's time were for or against the circulation. Many ignored it, and at least two of those who did so, Helkiah Crooke and Alexander Reade, knew Harvey and could have seen his demonstrations at the College of Physicians. But when their books appeared, Crooke's *Microcosmographia*, reprinted in 1631, and Reade's *Manuall of anatomy*, published in 1634, neither thought it necessary to make the slightest reference to the circulation. Perhaps it was because they were both concerned with the education of surgeons that they thought it imprudent to depart from the time-honoured Galenic doctrines and introduce any 'novelty' into their works. Even more surprising is it to find that one London surgeon could in 1630 still describe the three-chambered heart, and what is more imply that he had seen it in a dissection![27]

We do not know what Harvey himself may have said of the circulation of the blood in the Anatomical Lectures which he gave at the College of Physicians after the publication of *De motu cordis*, or even if he gave any. We do not at present know what his immediate successors had to say, nor who first publicly upheld the theory of the circulation in the College. In January 1648, however, it was the turn of Baldwin Hamey to give the *Prelectiones* and the manuscript of his lectures is still in the library of the College. His account of the heart and of the circulation of the blood is lengthy and detailed and is interspersed with learned references to the ancients, to Aristotle and Hippocrates, but most of all to Galen. He seems to be intent on reconciling the phenomenon of the circulation with Galenic theory, but at the same time is most careful to explain that it was entirely unknown to anyone before Harvey. He warns his audience that the meaning of the word 'circulation' as used by Harvey in an anatomical or physiological context, is totally different from its connotation in the ancient writings:

> ... now we truely know what ἐγκυκλοπαιδειά is, and what is meant by *Circularis Disciplina*, for it may be shew'd us in every body that hath a Heart: wherein we are more happy than they themselves that composed the word, who never pretended to so much knowledge in Anatomie,

as to frame a word by designe for our Art, though it serve our turne exactly by interpretation.

Though Hamey's lectures are interesting in themselves in that they show what experiments he had done and where his own interest in the subject principally lay, they add nothing of value to the subject and we would probably be wrong in supposing that all the ideas expressed in them met with Harvey's entire approval.

NOTES

1. British Museum, MS Sloane 1343; printed F. J. Cole, *J. Hist. Med.* XII (1957), 291–324. Quoted Keynes, *Life*, p. 319.
2. In *Epistolica exercitatio in qua principia philosophiae Rob. Fluddi reteguntur*, Paris 1630.
3. Anyone wishing to follow the controversy in detail may do so with the aid of the article by Dr E. Weil, 'An Echo of Harvey', *J. Hist. Med.*, XII (1957), pp. 167–74, or with the bibliography reproduced from this article in Keynes, *Life*, pp. 447–55. For an earlier discussion of the reception, see H. P. Bayon, 'William Harvey, Physician and Biologist', *Annals of Science*, III (1938), pp. 83–118.
4. The quotations which follow from Descartes are from the Pléiade edition, *Oeuvres et Lettres*, Paris 1953.
5. Mersenne, *Correspondence*, t. III, ed. Tanning & de Waard, Paris 1946, p. 346.
6. *Ibid.*, t. II, Paris 1945, p. 623.
7. 'Et, afin qu'on ait moins de difficulté à entendre ce que j'en dirai, je voudrais que ceux qui ne sont point versés en l'anatomie prissent la peine, avant que de lire ceci, de faire couper devant eux le coeur de quelque grand animal qui ait des poumons, car il est en tous assez semblable à celui de l'homme, et qu'ils fissent montrer les deux chambres ou concavités qui y sont . . . etc. (p. 158).
8. *Oeuvres*, ed. Adam et Tannery, t. XI, Paris 1909, p. 242.
9. That the blood acquired its colour from the liver was a commonly held belief whose truth Harvey denied by showing that the liver is different in colour in different animals. He concluded that the colour of the viscera depends on the colour of the blood. See *Lectures*, pp. 125, 143, 145, where he contradicts the views expressed by Laurentius in his *Historia anatomica*.
10. Quoted from an English version contained in a volume of letters and papers belonging to Dr Henry Power, British Museum, MS Sloane 1393.

11. Thomas Bartholin, *Epistolarum medicinalium a doctis vel ad doctos scriptarum*, Cent. I, Hagae Comitum, 1740, pp. 173–4.

12. See below p. 190.

13. In Beverwijk, *Epistolicae quaestiones cum doctorum responsis*, Rotterdam 1644, pp. 119–21.

14. Quoted by Keynes, *Life*, p. 321.

15. 'ut cum Chymistis loquar': *De Thorace*, Frankfurt 1627, Bk III, cap. 11, p. 95.

16. *Apologia pro Galeno*, Lyons 1668, cap. 55, p. 118.

17. *De thorace*, Bk II, cap. 23, p. 56.

18. 'Indeed, I find the whole idea absurd': *Apologia pro Galeno*, cap. 49, p. 108.

19. Both letters are quoted in translation in Keynes, *Life*, pp. 232–7, from the original paper by Ferrario, Poynter and Franklin in *J. Hist. Med.*, XV (1960), 7–21. The reader is warned that there are several errors in the translation.

20. As the text has not been reprinted since the seventeenth century, it will be found in the Appendix, together with a translation, pp. 238–47.

21. 'The demonstration that'.

22. Cf. a similar statement in the *Anatomical Lectures*, p. 101: 'Nature prefers things to be perfect, properly divided and done as well as may be. . . . Consequently Nature has ordained parts which are different and which come successively into action.'

23. 'William Harvey's conception of the heart as a pump', *Bull. Hist. Med.*, XXXIX, (1965) 508–17.

24. Quoted by G. V. Blackstone, *A History of the British Fire Service*, London 1957, p. 29.

25. Harvey uses this analogy also in the Second Letter to Riolan: '. . . you shall find all the strokes, order, vehemency, and intermission of the heart; just as you might feel in the palm of your hand water squirted through a syringe at divers and several shootings . . .' (pp. 149–50).

26. British Museum, MS Sloane 3306, f. 131.

27. 'There are in the heart three cells or ventricles, the one in the right side the other in the left and the third in the midst. . . . In the pitt of the middell ventricle [the blood] is digestid and purified. Then is itt sent unto the left ventricle where of the bloud is a spiritt engendred that is more pure and subtle then any bodye made of the foure elements.' From a treatise entitled 'Institution of the Anatomiae of man, 1630', in British Museum, MS Sloane 413. The author is named as Sam Sambrooke. A surgeon of this name was a member of the Company of Barber-Surgeons at this date and might have been the author. It will be remembered that this was also the surname of Harvey's apothecary mentioned by Aubrey.

Chapter Eight

The Debate with Riolan 1648–1649

IN 1649, Harvey published *Exercitationes duae anatomicae de circulatione sanguinis*. They were printed simultaneously in Cambridge and Rotterdam and were addressed to Jean Riolan the younger of Paris. Seeing that the judgement of posterity has been harsh on Riolan, finding him arrogant and a bitter controversialist and deeming his ideas on the circulation little short of preposterous, it has sometimes been wondered why Harvey should have chosen to answer him alone of all those who attacked *De motu cordis* or advanced alternative hypotheses. The reason would seem to be simply that Harvey and he were friends and that Riolan in his younger days had been an anatomist of outstanding ability. Harvey himself calls him the 'Prince of anatomists', and so too does Paul Marquand Slegel, who further praises him by saying, 'if anyone start to read all the anatomists without having read Riolan, he will miss many things that he should know; but if he read only the writings of Riolan and then, without reading any of the others, put his hand to dissection, he will become a great anatomist.'

Harvey refers directly to his friendship for Riolan in the letter which he wrote to Slegel in 1651: 'For the sake of the old friendship subsisting between us . . . and the high praise which he has lavished on the doctrine of the circulation, I cannot find it in my heart to say anything severe of Riolan.' There are two periods during which it seems likely that they met: the first in 1631, the second between 1638 and 1641. As is well known, Riolan was the personal physician to Queen Marie de Médicis, the widow of Henri IV, and mother of Louis XIII and Henrietta Maria, wife of Charles I. His connection with the French Court had already begun before 1628.[1] It was the time of the Religious Wars in France, and of plots and counter-plots centering on Marie de Médicis in her struggle to overthrow the dominance of Cardinal Richelieu and re-assert her own control over the young King, Louis XIII. In this she was unsuccessful, and in 1630 she was exiled from France and fled to Brussels. That Riolan was with her at the time is unlikely. Meantime, in England, Queen Henrietta Maria had successfully borne her second son, the future Charles II, on 29 May 1630. By the summer of 1631 she was again known to be pregnant and on 4 November, Mary, the future Princess of Orange, was born. On 22 August 1631, a passport was issued by the Secretary of State in the name of 'Dr Riolant'. It was issued in reply to a letter sent to Henrietta Maria by Madame Riolant asking for leave to return to France for herself, her two children and her husband, 'principal physician of the Queen's mother'. [2] On 12 April 1631, Riolan had given the public anatomy in the Faculté de Médicine in Paris, and, therefore, must have come to England after this date. He was back in Paris and attending meetings of the Faculté by October. [3] It is not unreasonable to suppose that he was sent to England by Marie de Médicis to attend her daughter, but why he should have left before the birth of the child is unknown. It is also strange that at this date he should be called 'principal physician' to the Queen's mother for the household accounts of Marie de Médicis do not refer to him. In 1631 her first physician was André du Chemin, [4] and it was only after his death in 1633 that Riolan succeeded to the office of first physician-in-ordinary to the Queen Mother. [5] In 1631, therefore, Riolan's attachment to her household can have been little more than nominal. The passport, however, indicates that he was in London and so could have met Harvey for the first time in this year.

After 1633, Riolan's attendance on Marie de Médicis was continuous until her death in 1642 in the house of Peter Paul Rubens in Cologne. Speaking of these years, Riolan explains how he found the charge a heavy one, for the never dared to leave the person of the Queen who was a valetudinarian. Consequently, he was forced to give up the practice of dissection, a thing he much regretted, and to absent himself from the Paris Faculté and his own library. Instead, he used the time to correct his earlier anatomical writings with a view to re-issuing them in a more correct and more complete form. From 18 October 1638 until 31 August 1641, Marie de Médicis was in England, and from what Riolan says about his attendance on her person there is little doubt that he was with her, although there is no known reference to his presence at the English Court. It is not impossible that the years which he spent in her service brought out the worst in Riolan's character and that under her influence his rather testy humour became soured and embittered. Marie de Médicis was a woman of limited intelligence and unlimited vanity. She was not a welcome guest in England and when, at last, she left there was a general expression of relief. As both Harvey and Riolan were about the Court in these years, we can assume that they met.

As a young man, Riolan had won for himself a reputation for precocious ability as an anatomist. He was born in Paris on 20 February 1580 and so was almost two years younger than Harvey. His father was Jean Riolan of Amiens, an eminent member and, for a period, Dean of the Faculty of Medicine of Paris, the author of several learned works including a text-book of anatomy. In 1602, the young Riolan was admitted Bachelor of Medicine in the University of Paris and in 1604, the year in which he took his doctorate, was appointed by Henri IV to the Regius chair of Anatomy and Pharmacy in that university. Four years later, in 1608, his first important anatomical work was published, *Schola anatomica novis et raris observationibus illustrata cui adiuncta est accurata foetus humani historia*.[6] In this book Riolan claims to have read all the anatomists and compared their works, and to have taken from them, with full acknowledgement, only those things which are true. The truth of these statements he has verified by dissection, for dissection is more useful to anatomy than long reading and deep meditation. So nothing will be found in this book which he has not personally verified in the human body. That this is no vain boast is evident. He was a man of outstanding erudition as is plain from every page, in which references to the classical writers and philosophers and to the Scriptures jostle with those to the medical writers of classical and Arabian antiquity and with allusions to the anatomists his contemporaries and immediate predecessors. There seems little doubt that for book learning he was unequalled among his contemporaries in France. But for all its learning, this book is not merely a rehash of ancient authority; it is, as Riolan justly claims, founded on his own numerous dissections and anatomical observations. It is true that he adheres strictly to Galen's precepts, but within this framework he controls and verifies theories by his own observations and does not spend time in idle speculation. The book was reprinted two years later under a new title, *Anatome corporis humani*. It contained more new discoveries but, contrary to what might have been expected from the reputation which posterity has given him, these discoveries are not eagerly claimed by Riolan,

177

but hidden in the body of the text and no particular stress laid upon them. He was to spend the next forty-five years in re-writing and re-editing versions of this *Anatome*, and as his knowledge of the subject improved and increased, so did this new knowledge become incorporated in his book. In 1618, the book underwent a complete revision and was republished under the title of *Anatomia seu anthropographia*. There, in the Foreword to the Reader, Riolan explains that he has seen many things which are contrary to the opinion of the younger anatomists, but he should not therefore be thought vain and mendacious, for opinion should only gain credence when dissection bears it out. Use and experience are the chief masters in the art of anatomy. His book is not to be regarded as the end of all knowledge on the subject, but merely as a help and guide. No man will be perfect in the art of anatomy simply by reading his book; he will have to read other books, to dissect and to practise. In 1626, the second and much enlarged edition of the *Anthropographia* was published, and it was from this edition that Harvey made the notes which he added to his own Anatomical Lectures. With many of the sentiments expressed by Riolan in the Foreword, he was totally in agreement.

The publication of anatomical writings was not the only kind of work on which Riolan was engaged in these years. He was assiduous in his attendance at the Faculté de Médicine, actively engaged in participation in its administrative and academic affairs, in teaching and in examining. He had written separate treatises on osteology, on giants and hermaphrodites, and had been a prime mover in the establishment in Paris of a permanent anatomical theatre and a botanical garden. Whatever he became later, Riolan had in his younger days an open and receptive mind, and, though a staunch defender of orthodox medicine and of Galen, did not allow the opinions of authority to outweigh evidence provided by dissection. Perhaps the main difference between him and Harvey in his youth was that he took more interest in anatomical structure than in function.

When Riolan returned to Paris in 1642, after the death of Marie de Médicis, he was a sick man, no longer capable of taking so active a part in the affairs of the Faculté. Already in October 1640, he had returned from London for an operation for the removal of a stone from the bladder. 'The operation was performed yesterday', wrote Guy Patin on 6 October, 'with doubtful success to judge by certain signs which have since appeared.' He was in Paris again briefly in May 1641 and on

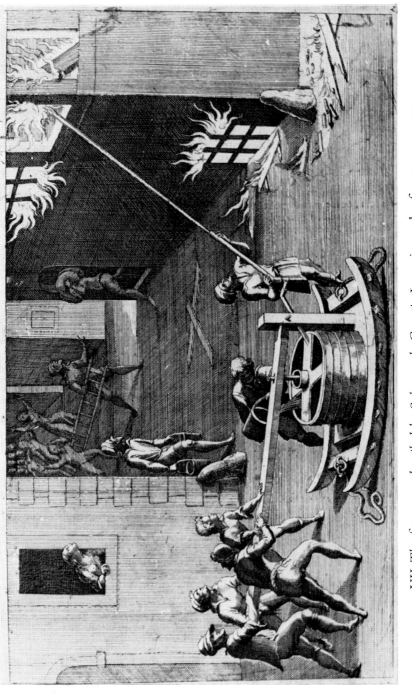

VII The fire-pump described by Salomon de Caus in Les raisons des forces mouvantes

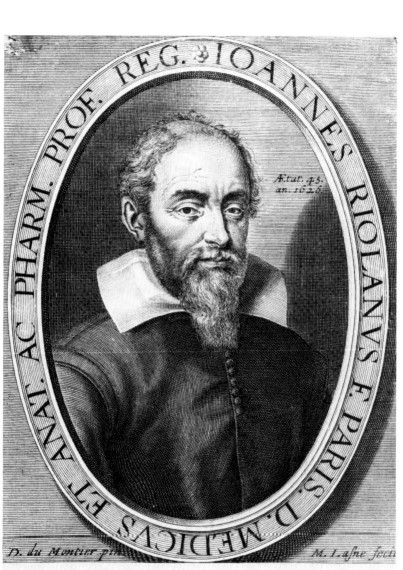

REG. ✿ IOANNES RIOLANVS F. PARIS D. MEDICVS ET ANAT. AC PHARM. PROF.

Ætat. 45.
an. 1626

D. du Montier pin.   M. Lasne fecit.

Cum me Phœbus amet, Phœbo sua semper apud me
Munera sunt Ossa, et suaue rubens Hyacinthus.

VIII Jean Riolan in 1626

this occasion Guy Patin remarks on his being soured by the little attention paid to his writings. In October of that year he underwent a second operation in Paris for the removal of more stones. By 1648 he was suffering from severe asthma and in 1654 near blindness was added to his miseries, and he gave up the Regius chair to his friend, Guy Patin. He died at the age of 77 on 19 February 1657, a few months before Harvey. His family circumstances in his latter years were far from happy and it is not altogether surprising that he became soured and embittered. It is only a pity that he is remembered for what he became rather than for what he had been, a brilliant teacher of anatomy who spoke with clarity, facility and erudition, a walking encyclopaedia of knowledge, the discoverer of a number of new things in anatomy and a man who believed that the value of ocular demonstration outweighed all the opinions of the ancients.[7]

The first official reference in the University of Paris to the circulation of the blood came in December 1642 when a disputation on the subject was held in the schools. Riolan was not present on that occasion and the conclusion reached was that the blood did indeed move in a circle. On 7 February 1645, however, another disputation was held, this time on the proposition 'Whether on account of the circulation of the blood Galen's *Methodus medendi* should be altered'. Riolan presided and for the first time, as far as is known, expounded his own theory of the circulation from which he concluded that Galen's Method did not have to be altered.

He begins by extolling the heart and exploiting to the full the analogy of the heart with the sun. He then speaks of the motive or pulsific faculty which the heart requires to fulfil its office, of its rhythmical movements in systole and diastole. Its perpetual movement requires an agent; as in pneumatic and hydraulic engines, so in the heart it is blood and air passing through the cavities which gives this perpetual movement in order to conserve the native heat of the heart and provide the body with nourishment. The blood, he says, is brought through the vena cava into the right sinus of the heart and from there the thicker part is carried through the pulmonary artery to the lungs for their nourishment, and returns to the vena cava by revulsion; the thinner part slips through the immobile but pervious septum into the left ventricle where it is converted into arterial blood and from thence conveyed to the limbs. Through the anastomoses between veins and arteries, this bloods seeps into the veins and so returns again to the heart as to its fount and origin, after the fashion of waters which mount up until they are level with their source. Truly, he continues, this circulation does not occur throughout the body two or three times a day, or once in an hour 'as some of the bolder assert', for both opinions are absurd and impossible. He believes it to vary in accordance with the state of health of the body, with the amount of food taken and excrement voided, and in healthy bodies to happen only once or twice a day. And moreover, seeing the continuity of the vena cava, the blood in the smaller vessels does not return to the heart unless it be forcibly recalled by a sudden lack of blood in the vena cava or aorta, or, propelled by some excitement, it leaves its own receptacles and rushes into the vena cava. In a pregnant woman, the blood of the foetus all returns to the heart of the mother until the foetal heart is perfected, at which time it has its own blood supply, as is proved by the impossibility of extracting a living foetus from a woman who has died. By this explanation of the movement of the blood, the medicine of Galen can be preserved. The liver is the instrument for the preparation of nutritive, venous blood imbued with natural spirit. There are two kinds of blood, venous and arterial, and they have different movements. Finally, he concludes with remarks on the treatment of various diseases. The exposition of his theory here is not a model of clarity. It is followed by twenty-nine objections, each of which is refuted in turn. In some of these mention is made of Harvey, and Riolan expresses his agreement with Harvey's view that the blood returns to the heart through the veins while at the same time upholding his own belief that there is no circulation through the portal vein. In everything that Riolan wrote on the subject of the circulation he invariably gave to Harvey the credit for being its discoverer.

Three years later, in 1648, Riolan published his *Encheiridium anatomicum et pathologicum*.[8] The novelty of this book lies in the fact that after discussing the anatomy of each part, Riolan adds a section on the diseases to which it is subject, their causes and so forth, and on the pathology of each part. In Bk III, cap. 8, he comes to the discussion of the heart and so writes his views on the circulation of the blood.

> The perpetual movement of the heart depends indeed on its innate faculty but it could not for long endure did not the blood arrive continually, the blood out of which the heart makes the vital spirit. Now, if in each pulsation the heart admits one or two drops of blood and drives out as much into the aorta, and if in the space of one hour it beats 2,000 times, it follows of necessity that a great part of the blood, or all of it

must pass through the heart in twelve or fifteen hours.[9] Now the quantity of blood contained in the vessels may be as much as 15 or 20 lb, and so this blood needs must pass two or three times through the heart in the space of twenty-four hours, according as to whether the heart's movement is faster or slower.

That this circulatory movement may be more easily and more conveniently maintained, William Harvey, Englishman, Royal Physician, and author and discoverer of this movement of the blood, and John Waleus, professor of Leyden, who defends and vigorously upholds it, believe the blood to be taken through the lungs from the right to the left ventricle of the heart and deny its passage through the septum of the heart, and so they believe that in one or two hours all the blood passes through the heart and through the whole body.[10] This I do not admit. . . .

When I consider the trunk of the vena cava, separated from the liver and continuous from the neck to the sacrum and nowhere interrupted nor passing through the liver, as is plainly to be seen and can be understood by inserting a probe, I am led to believe that the vena cava originates from the heart as the portal vein from the liver, and that these two veins have quite different blood in them, albeit both kinds are elaborated in the liver, one kind which is entrusted to the portal vein, the other which is carried to the heart through a branch which arises from the liver and which is twice as small as the trunk of the vena cava.

The blood which is contained in the portal vein does not circulate, although it has a flux and reflux within its receptacles and communicates with the coeliac arteries which are joined to each other by their mutual anastomoses. Within those vessels the blood can have a reciprocal ebb and flow, but it does not go out through the whole length of the body and it is not circulated.

And therefore, the circulation which occurs in the heart takes for its use material from the liver through the vena cava. The circulatory vessels are the aorta and the vena cava, but their offshoots have no part in that circulation, because, when the blood is poured out into all the parts of the second and third region, it remains there to nourish them and does not flow back to the greater vessels unless it is drawn back by force, when there is a great lack of blood in the larger vessels, or driven back by impulsion or frenzy into the greater circulatory vessels.

And so the blood brought from the liver to the right ventricle of the heart passes through the septum into the left ventricle. I do not deny that when the circulation is violent, the blood may be carried through the lungs to the left ventricle where it is sent out headlong into the aorta so that afterwards it may be transferred into the larger veins of the joints, veins which communicate with the arteries by mutual anastomoses.

Then by the veins it goes back upwards to the right ventricle of the heart, and thus is accomplished the circulation by continuous flux and reflux of the blood. Just as the blood of the veins perpetually and naturally ascends or returns to the heart, so the blood of the arteries descends or goes away from the heart. Nevertheless, if the small veins of the arms and legs were to become emptied, the blood of the veins can go down into them to fill up the vacant space, as I have clearly demonstrated against Harvey and Waleus.

No one can deny the mutual anastomoses of the veins and arteries seeing that Galen described this very thing, demonstrated it experimentally, and everyday experience confirms it. Hippocrates himself, in *De articulis*, Bk III, promises a separate work on the communications, κοινωνίας, of veins and arteries.

You see how great is the need of circulated blood for the continual motion of the heart, and in what manner the circulation occurs without confusion and perturbation of the humours and destruction of the ancient medicine.

The circulation of the blood is as necessary for the continued movement of the heart as in mills is the stream of water which flows over the wheels and drives their revolution; it is necessary in order that the blood which is impoverished by the casting forth of spirits wheresoever it goes may be re-heated and re-invigorated and acquire new spirits in the heart; and in order also that the heart which is the source of native heat may be perpetually moistened with drops of liquid so that it does not burn up, which would happen if this dewy liquid failed, or, as I will call it with Louis Duret, this συῤῥόης or nectar of life were insufficient.

Riolan's opinion on the blood's movement seems to have arisen from his attempt to reconcile strict Galenic belief with Harvey's theory of the circulation. The resulting inconsistencies and contradictions Harvey was not slow to point out. Indeed so little of either truth or sense is there in the whole passage, that one can only admire Harvey's patience in his reply. What is abundantly clear from the passage is that Riolan is theorising without looking, and his theorising is dictated by his passionate desire to see the medicine of Galen kept intact and his fear lest Harvey's doctrine overturn its foundations. It was this emotional attitude to the subject which blinded his eyesight and clouded his judgement.

Harvey's First Letter to Riolan is a direct criticism of the *Encheiridium*. It is not a general discussion of the circulation, but treats only of the points raised by Riolan. Harvey was fully aware of the reasons for which Riolan had got himself into this tangle, partly admitting and partly denying the circulation 'and why he endeavours to build a reeling and tottering opinion of the Circulation: Lest, forsooth, he should destroy the antient rules of Physick' (p. 124).[11] Harvey's aim in his First Letter, then, is twofold: to refute Riolan on every point and to show that his own doctrine of the total circulation of the blood does not destroy the ancient physic but further it.

He begins by pointing out the contradictions which are to be found in Riolan's *Encheiridium* as a result of his statement that the blood does not circulate in the derivatives of the vena cava. If the coeliac and mesenteric arteries do, by his own admission, bring in blood at every pulsation, this blood must go out through the portal vein, or the portal vein will burst. Mere ebb and flow in it would serve no purpose, and the blood cannot go backwards against the force of the influx. To Riolan's argument that there are no valves in the mesentery to prevent the regress of blood, like the sigmoids of the heart, Harvey answers that they exist in the splenic branch, and in those deep veins in which they are not found their presence is not required, for the action of the muscles is sufficient to drive the blood towards the heart and prevent its return.[12] He calculates the amount of blood entering the mesentery by comparison with that which can be shown to enter the arm by the experiment of the ligature. As the mesenteric arteries are greater than those of the carpus, the force of blood entering it must needs be greater. If Riolan will only consider the force with which blood leaps out of a cut artery, 'as if it were shot out of a spout',

> I think he would scarce believe that any part of blood which only enters could against this impulsion and influx pass back again, being not able to drive it back with force. For which cause, considering these things with himself, I believe it would not even enter his mind to imagin that the blood out of the veins of the *porta* could creep back by these same ways; and so disburthen it self into the Mesenterie, against so forcible and strong an influx into the arteries (p. 128).

Harvey then points out that by saying that some blood needs circular motion, and this the venous blood in the vena cava, while the venous blood in the portal vein does not, Riolan is implying that there are two kinds of blood in these vessels, and this does not appear to be the case nor does Riolan prove it to be so. He then attacks Riolan's contention that the lacteal vessels carry chyle to the liver, where it is

183

changed into blood and from thence carried to the left ventricle of the heart and asks how this can be, seeing that Riolan denies that the blood from the portal vein passes through the liver. He then quotes Riolan's statement to the effect that blood in the arteries naturally descends from the heart, whereas that in the veins returns to it, saying that if Riolan really believed it he would have no difficulty about the movement of chyle, for the old belief that blood moved one way in the portal vein and chyle the other would be ended. The mesenteric veins suck the chyle from the intestines and carry it to the liver. This is obvious in a chick embryo and it follows that it also happens in an adult. With this Harvey dismisses all further discourse of the lacteals saying that he will give his views concerning them in another place.[13]

Harvey now turns to Riolan's opinion that, in the branches of the vena cava and of the aorta in the second and third regions, there is no circulation because the blood is used up by the parts for their nourishment. In reply to this Harvey has two points to make. First, although some part of the blood must be assimilated if it is to nourish the part,

> it is not needful, that the whole influx should remain there for the conversion of so little a portion; for every part does not use so much blood for its nourishment, as it contains in its veins, arteries and porosities... (p. 131).

Second, that Riolan actually contradicts this opinion when he speaks of the brain sending back blood to cool the heart. This Harvey says is paralleled in cases of fever where the patient throws off his clothes in an effort to cool the blood which thus cooled returns to cool the heart.

> Whence the most learned man seems to insinuate a kind of necessity, that as from the brain, so there is a circulation from all the parts, otherwise than before he had openly declared (p. 132).

Harvey then repeats yet once again his own views on the propulsion of blood through the arteries and its return through the veins. It is interesting to notice what he has to say here on the way in which the blood passes from the arteries into the veins. He seems to think that the blood from the extreme ends of the arteries is extravasated into the tissues and forced by the pressure of blood behind, and by the action of the muscles and joints and of the parts, into the extreme ends of the veins:

Besides that, the blood which is contained in all parts of the second and third region, by the force of the blood directed and driven by every pulse, is forced out of the pores into the veins, out of the branches into the greater vessels, as likewise by the motion and compression of the parts adjacent; for that which is contained is thrust out by every thing containing it, when it is pressed and streightned: so by the motion of muscles and the joynts, the branches of the veins passing between, being pressed and streightned, thrust the blood contained in the lesser vessels into the greater (p. 133).

It is an explanation which he had not given in his letter to Hofmann in 1636 and it is different from the account that he was to give in 1651 to Slegel, where he explains his idea of anastomoses. Both explanations remained for him unverifiable.

Having said that Riolan agrees with him that the systole of the heart causes the diastole of the arteries, and that the blood cannot return to the heart from the arteries because of the valves, he points out that this necessitates a belief that the arteries pulsate to their very tips. The use of the circulation, then, is to warm the body and Riolan is wrong in wishing to deprive any part of this benefit. Here there is nothing different from what he had already said in De motu cordis, but the muddled thinking of Riolan provokes him to write:

> For which cause most learned *Riolan* seems to me, when he says, that in some parts there is no Circulation, to speak rather officiously [*sc.* expediently], than truth; to wit, that he might please most men, and oppose nobody, and that he rather wrote humanely, than gravely, in the behalf of truth (p. 136).

This he says Riolan does when he denies the pulmonary transit of the blood, preferring to believe that it goes through 'uncertain and hidden passages' in the septum, rather than through the wide-open vessels of the lungs. Again, he points to inconsistencies in Riolan's statements concerning the lungs elsewhere in the same book. Riolan could clearly not make up his mind about the pulmonary transit and Harvey furnishes no proofs of its existence and no arguments to support it beyond the general certainty of its truth from his own experimental proofs of the general circulation. Having quoted Riolan's remarks to the effect that if the pulmonary transit exists, then there are two circulations, a pulmonary and a general, Harvey adds a description of the coronary circulation. This he had not mentioned in De motu cordis, for indeed it follows from the general, but it is the shortest in the body.

185

The most learned man in this place might have added the third circulation, which is a very short one, out of the left ventricle into the right, drawing about a part of the blood through the coronall arteries and veins, by its branches, which are distributed about the bodie, walls, and septum of the heart (p. 138).

With masterly clarity Harvey sums up all the inconsistencies in Riolan's opinion[14] and tries to persuade him that if he believes in a partial circulation he must in fact believe in the total. He concludes with an attack on Riolan's belief in anastomoses and here describes the only experiment to be mentioned in this Letter. In spite of his search for anastomoses, Harvey says that he has never found anything at all like them except in the choroid plexus, in the vascular system of the testicle and in the umbilical arteries whose terminal threads are 'obliterated' in the coats of the umbilical veins. That they nowhere exist he proves as follows:

Opening the breast of any creature, and tying the *vena cava* near the heart so that nothing can pass that way into the heart, and presently cutting the neck arteries, not touching the veins on either side. If by giving vent [*sc.* making an incision] you see the arteries emptied, and not the veins too, I hope it will be clear that the blood is carried out of the veins into the arteries, no where but through the ventricles of the heart: Otherwise (as *Galen* has observ'd) in a little space we should see the veins emptyed, and destitute of blood by the efflux of the arteries (pp.143–4).

The Second Letter to Riolan partakes of a totally different character from the First. Though Harvey addresses Riolan in the first sentence, he makes no mention of him throughout the Letter and only in the final paragraph does he turn to two specific points in Riolan's opinion on the circulation, his denial that blood circulates through the portal vein and his belief in arterio-venous anastomoses, to refute both by experimental evidence. The same quality of elegant simplicity which characterises all Harvey's experiments in *De motu cordis* is to be seen in his demonstration of the portal circulation:

I will conclude (most learned *Riolan*) to give you more ample satisfaction, because you think that there is no Circulation in the mesentericks: Let the *vena porta* be tied near to the *cymus* [*sc.* the central sphere] of the liver in a live dissection which you may easily try, you shall see by the swelling of the veins beneath the ligature, that same come to pass which happens in blood-letting by tying of the left arm, which will show you the passage of the blood there (pp. 192–3).

186

The experiment designed to dispose of the idea of the existence of arterio-venous anastomoses is similar to that described in the First Letter but concerns different vessels, thus confirming the belief that Harvey must have searched for anastomoses many times and tried to find them experimentally in all the different parts of the body. To deny the existence of anastomoses in the Galenic sense, that is the conjunction of veins and arteries by wide-mouthed osculations in their contiguous sides through which arterial and venous blood could pass indifferently in either direction, was vital to Harvey's whole theory of the circulation; but, paradoxically, the existence of a one-way connection between arteries and veins was essential to this theory. Although Harvey speaks here and there of transudation into tissues, it seems as though the intimate connection between blood and tissue that is required for its nutrition was never clearly defined in his thought. Though these experiments in the Letters to Riolan prove that anastomoses in the Galenic sense do not exist, Harvey does not here explain in any detail how he thinks the transference of blood from the arteries to the veins does occur. As has already been said, this explanation will be found in his letter to Slegel written in 1651.

> And when you shall hear any man of that opinion, that by *Anastomosis* the blood can come out of the veins into the arteries, tie in a live dissection the great vein [*sc.* the vena cava], near the division of the crurals, and as soon as you cut the artery (because it finds passage) you shall see all the mass of blood emptied out of all the veins (nay, out of the ascendent *cava* too) by the pulse of the heart, in a very short time, yet that below the ligature the crural veins and parts below are only full. Which, if it could any way have returned into the arteries by an *Anastomosis*, should never have come to passe (p. 193).

The greater part of Harvey's Second Letter is a restatement of his hypothesis concerning the circulation of the blood, supported by further experimental proof. Riolan's thesis had been completely and satisfactorily demolished in the First Letter and the Second is not concerned to answer him. If we ask why Harvey should then have written two Letters to Riolan, the answer is perhaps that Riolan merely provided the excuse for the publication of the Second Letter, that Harvey had already written it before he received Riolan's *Encheiridium* and that he had written it for all those who attacked his hypothesis. It was convenient to put the two Letters together between the covers of one book. By adding Riolan's name at the beginning and the final paragraph of

187

experimental refutation, it could be made relevant. That it was designed as a supplement to *De motu cordis* is clear from what Harvey says about it in the introductory paragraphs:

> In my book concerning the motion of the heart and blood in creatures, I only chose out those things out of my many other observations, by which I either thought that errours were confuted, or truth was confirm'd; I left out many things as unnecessary and unprofitable, which notwithstanding are discernible by dissection and sense; of which I shall now add some in few words, in favour of those that desire to learn (p. 147).

It is much closer in style to *De motu cordis* than is the First Letter where Harvey is arguing dialectically and not experimentally. The Second Letter is concerned to affirm a truth and prove its validity by arguments drawn from experimental evidence, not to deny a falsity. Its style is more incisive and more direct, and it seems to flow with greater ease, without repetitions and turnings around the same point. As it is difficult to find any logical basis in Riolan's statements in the *Encheiridium*, so it is difficult to find any logical continuity or coherence in Harvey's criticisms. The Second Letter falls into a number of obvious chapters or divisions. It begins with further proofs that the propulsion of the blood through the arteries is caused by the heart. It then discusses what differences, if any, there are between venous and arterial blood and so goes on to a general discourse on the subject of spirits. It then returns to the propulsion of the blood by the heart and moves on to the question of the final cause of the circulation. It returns to the movement of the blood in the veins and in the arteries and to the question of the heart's action, and this passage ends with a brief résumé of the circulation. The final remarks concern the flow of blood in the veins, and the question of transfusion from arteries to veins, Descartes's opinion of systole and diastole, which is refuted, the necessity for the circulation and its clinical implications. This analysis shows that the argument is not as tightly worked out as in *De motu cordis* but weaves around one basic theme, the movement of blood in the arteries and veins, its immediate cause and its manner. This Second Letter, however, should not be considered as merely a supplement to *De motu cordis*. The points discussed in it are chosen to answer specific criticisms or to refute alternative notions. In so far as it is an answer to any one person in particular, it might be taken as an answer to Descartes, though he was not alone in holding some of the views here shown to be incompatible with experimental observation.

Harvey begins his Letter by saying that scarcely a day has passed since the publication of *De motu cordis* without some good or evil being said about the circulation. He has been subjected to much scurrilous invective.

> But I think it a thing unworthy of a Philosopher and a searcher of the truth, to return bad words for bad words; and I think I shall doe better and more advised, if with the light of true and evident observations I shall wipe away those symptomes of incivility (p. 146).

From these writings nothing of good can come and he has not troubled to read them; but for those who want to learn without railing against his vivisections and animal investigations, and who realise that even in the meanest creatures 'the great and Almighty Father is sometimes most conspicuous', he will add more proofs of the circulation.

The first experiment designed to prove that the pulse in the arteries is produced by the force of the blood driven into them from the heart, is a repetition of Galen's experiment with a hollow reed, the experiment which Harvey had termed impossible in his Lectures and in *De motu cordis*. Though Galen and Vesalius had both referred to it, neither, Harvey says, had tried it, and he adds that in any case it would have been useless for them, for it shows the presence of the arterial pulse beyond the reed and so proves that it cannot be conveyed through the coats of the artery. He likens the experiment to the findings which he had already noted in *De motu cordis* concerning the pulsating aneurism, and in further confirmation relates the case of a nobleman whose descending aorta was found on post-mortem examination to be calcified, yet who, in life, had a very evident pulsation in his feet and legs, a thing which could not have happened did the arterial pulse proceed from the arterial coats. In this section, Harvey also suggests the performance of the simple experiment of dividing an artery and putting a finger over the cut. The blood will be noticed coming down the artery and dilating it at each contraction of the heart. If the finger be lifted, the blood will spurt out through the cut at each contraction of the heart and it will be seen that it reflects the rhythm, order, intermission and force of the heart beat, like water squirted out through a syringe.[15] The section ends with remarks on the contraction of the arteries which Harvey ascribes to a power inherent in their coats, because their systole is their return from distension to their natural state.

> ... they are not dilated and streightned for the same cause, nor by the same instrument, but by severall [*sc.* different], as you may observe in the motion of all the parts, and in the heart; it is distended by the ear, contracted by it self, so the arteries are dilated by the heart and fall of themselves (pp. 151–2).

Harvey now turns to discuss the differences between arterial and venous blood. He suggests the experiment of drawing off a quantity of each kind into two separate bowls and allowing both to clot, upon which he says it will be immediately obvious whether or not there is any difference. Though this is not a crucial experiment, Harvey thought that it showed what he believed, that arterial blood was not more 'spiritous' than venous. It is in what he says about the alleged differences between the two kinds of blood that he seems to have the criticism of Descartes in mind:

> they do ascribe to the arteries a fresher sort of blood, of a more florid colour, more frothy, and imbued with an abundance of I know not what spirits, effervescing and swelling, and occupying a greater space, like milk or honey set upon the fire. [16]

If one drop of blood from the left ventricle did thus ferment and distend the whole aorta, on cooling it would return to its natural size, but as this does not happen in the bowl of cold arterial blood which behaves exactly like the cold venous blood, there cannot be this difference between them.

> Sense and reason alike assure us that the blood contained in the left ventricle is not of a different nature from that in the right.

He then examines the three reasons for this belief in diversity. He attributes the observed difference in colour to the effect of what he calls 'straining'. Through a small orifice only the thinner and lighter part of the blood escapes and the thicker, over which the thinner part swims, is left behind, but out of a large orifice it comes all together in a great stream. So the difference in colour in the blood in the lungs is ascribed by him to the 'straining' effect of the pulmonary tissues. He is far from thinking that it is the air in the lungs which has anything to do with the colour of the blood. The emptiness of the arteries and of the left ventricle in a dead dissection he correctly ascribes to the fact that the heart continues to beat after the lungs have collapsed, for in those who die as a result of the simultaneous collapse of the lungs and cessation of the heart beat, as for instance in drowning, both the veins and arteries will be found full of blood. It was, doubtless, this finding of empty arteries that had led Erasistratus to the belief that they contained nothing but aerial spirits.

At this point Harvey digresses into a discussion of these spirits, a topic which he had carefully avoided in *De motu cordis*.

> As concerning . . . the Spirits, what they are, and of what consistence, and how they are in the body, whether they be apart and distinct from the solid parts, or mix'd with them, there are so many and so diverse opinions that it is no wonder if Spirits, whose nature is left so doubtfull, do serve for a common escape to ignorance: For commonly ignorant persons when they cannot give a reason for any thing, they say presently, that it is done by Spirits, and bring in Spirits as performers in all cases; and like as bad Poets do bring in the gods upon the Scene by head and ears, to make the *Exit* and *Catastrophe* of their play (p. 155).

Fernel, having found empty 'cells' in the brain thought them to be full of spirits since Nature abhors a vacuum. The physicians believe in natural spirits in the veins, vital spirits in the arteries and animal spirits in the nerves.

> But none of these have we found by dissection, neither in the veins, nerves, arteries, nor parts of living persons (p. 156).

Some think these spirits are corporeal, others incorporeal:

> and those who make corporeal Spirits, sometimes say, that the blood or thinnest part of the blood, is the conjunction of the soul with the body; sometimes they say, that the Spirits are contained in the blood (as flame in smoke) and sustain'd by the perpetuall flux of it; sometimes they do distinguish them from the blood (p. 156).

Those who believe in incorporeal spirits are in even greater difficulties for their notions get confused with the philosophical ideas on potential spirits, concoctive spirits, procreative spirits, and so forth, where spirits are confused with faculties. Another complication derives from the scholastic and theological opinions of spirits of good and evil. And 'although there is nothing more uncertain and doubtfull than the doctrine which is assign'd [*sc.* proposed] to us concerning the spirits, yet most physicians follow Hippocrates in believing the body to be made up of three parts, namely that which contains, that which is contained and that which causes action, by which spirits are understood.' By this, of course, Harvey means 'motive spirit', the power which

191

makes movement of all kinds possible, and he concludes that if this definition be accepted, then anything which causes any kind of activity in the human body must be 'spirit'.

That this is in fact his own opinion on 'spirit' is clear from what he says on the specific problem of the spirit in the blood. As this whole question will be discussed later in connection with *De generatione*,[17] it will be sufficient here merely to summarise what Harvey has written. Spirit cannot be separated from blood any more than flame from fire or spirits of wine from wine. So the spirit which inheres in arterial blood is either its act or its agent. It does not cause the blood to swell or ferment as is shown by the experiment with the bowls of arterial and venous blood; in this respect arterial and venous blood are the same, though perhaps arterial blood may be possessed of a higher quantity of spirit than venous blood. Neither the animal, nor the natural, nor the vital spirits are to be thought of as 'divers sorts of vapours' (p. 158). If they are thought of as vapours, how do they pass through the body, independently of the blood, or inherently connected with it? If they exist as an exhalation of the blood, like steam, then they pass with the blood wherever it goes; they are not distinct from the blood on which they depend for their existence and from which they are perpetually vanishing, and so 'they neither flow back nor pass away, nor abide [*sc.* remain at rest], but according to the influxion, refluxion, or passing of the blood, as being either their subject, *vehiculum*, or nourishment' (p. 158). Those who think that the spirits are created in the heart from a mixture of inspired air and an exhalation from the blood, caused either by the innate heat of the heart or its motion,[18] are postulating the existence of something which is colder than the heart and colder than the blood and therefore must derive its heat from the blood and not itself be the agent for warming the blood. 'Such Spirits are rather to be deem'd fumes and excrements, flowing from the blood and body (like smels), than workers in Nature; especially since they being so frail and vanishing, do so quickly lose that vertue, which in their original they receive from the blood' (p. 159). Harvey brings the long digression to an end with a taunt at those who expatiate on the virtue of innate heat as the preserver of life and ascribe its means of action to spirits, but do not realise that its means of action is blood.[19]

Harvey resumes the discussion of the passage of blood through the arteries and veins with the description of the simple experiment of cutting a vein and artery and watching the blood pour out from the distal side of a cut vein and squirt out, 'as if it were out of a spout', from the central side of a severed artery. So the direction of the flow of blood in both sets of vessels is immediately obvious. What is more, the blood moves with velocity in a continuous flow, not drop by drop. To prove that no air is contained, plunge the severed orifice of vein and artery in water, and were any air therein, bubbles would immediately betray its presence. Air blown into the veins from the heart towards the extremities, cannot pass the valves, much less can the blood.[20] And so it is certain that the blood does not leave the heart through the veins. And that this movement of the blood is continually going on in the living body is proved by the action of the heart which perpetually drives out the blood at every stroke. Only when the heart is so excessively distended that it cannot admit any more blood does it cease to beat and death from asphyxia follows 'as we have seen in the Anatomie of living creatures'; the arteries continue to receive the blood driven into them in great quantity. It would seem that Harvey is here alluding to the opinion, held by Descartes, that the blood enters the arteries only drop by drop.

Harvey now restates his opinion that the efficient cause of the circulation is the motion of the heart and refers to his discussion of this point in *De motu cordis*. He then concludes that it is the contractile element in muscle which endows the heart with its capacity for movement, a conclusion which is, however, rather inferred than stated. He then turns to those who reject the whole hypothesis of the circulation because they understand neither its efficient nor its final cause. Here he plainly says that until the fact of the circulation be generally accepted, it is useless to enquire for what purpose it was designed, an opinion he had already expressed in his letter to Hofmann.

> And first I own I am of opinion that our first duty is to inquire whether the thing be or not, before asking wherefore it is? for from the fact and circumstances which meet us when the circulation is admitted and established, the ends and objects of its institution are especially to be sought.[21]

The circulation is not to be rejected because it does not explain everything, or because it upsets preconceived notions:

> the deeds of nature, which are manifest to the sense, care not for any opinion or any antiquity, for there is nothing more antient than nature, or of greater authority (p. 166).

193

With some speculations on the probability that the circulation of the blood through the body is not the same at all times or in all places, Harvey leaves conjecture to return to yet further experimental proofs that the arterial pulse is caused by the impulse of the blood.

To demonstrate this, Harvey recommends that a length of animal's gut be taken, filled with water and tied at both ends. If it is then tapped at one end, the vibration will be felt at the other. In this same manner the physician can distinguish between abdominal ascites due to fluid and tympanites caused by the presence of flatus. This experiment, Harvey points out, is one which raised the most formidable objection to his hypothesis of the circulation, but an objection which no one had thought of. The systole and diastole of the pulse can, in this demonstration, be simulated without the escape of any fluid. (This is not a real difficulty. In Harvey's model there is transmission of a pulse wave, but no forward movement of the fluid. These two things can be distinguished in the arteries where the movement of the blood takes place but is much slower than the velocity of the pulse wave.) However, as the auricles fill the ventricles and the ventricles the arteries, and because valves prevent the return of blood, this state of affairs cannot exist in the body, for the arteries must pass on the blood or burst, or the heart be suffocated by over distention. This has already been sufficiently proved in *De motu cordis* by the vivisection of snakes. In further confirmation of this, Harvey recounts the experiment which he performed in the presence of King Charles I:

> In the internal jugular vein of a live Doe, which I laid open before a great part of the Nobility, and the King my Royal Master standing by, which was cut and broke off in the middle: From the lower part rising from the Clavicule, scarce a few drops did issue, whilst in the mean time the blood with great force, and breaking out of a round stream, ran out most plentifully downwards from the head through the other orifice of the vein (p. 170).

The daily experience of phlebotomy shows that the blood emerges from the distal side of the cut vein and that its flow can be impeded by pressure with the finger below the cut. Further experiments to show the direction of the venous blood flow follow, and remarks on hyperemia resulting from venous occlusion. To emphasise the force of the blood flow in the body, Harvey cites the case of Sir Robert Darcy[22] whose left ventricle was found on post-mortem inspection to have been ruptured as a result of an impediment which prevented the flow of blood from the left ventricle into the arteries. From this and other post-mortem findings, Harvey concludes that

> Although . . . there may be an impulsion without an exite [as in the experiment with the water in the gut], . . . yet cannot it be so in the blood which is in the vessels of living persons, without very great and heavy impediments and dangers (pp. 173-4).

The next point which Harvey discusses concerns the variations which can occur in the circulation in different parts of the body, in different circumstances and at different times of life. After this comes a digression in which Harvey expresses his opinion of those who try to refute anatomical evidence with far-fetched argument, and he quotes Aristotle and Plato in his own support: if things demonstrated are perceptible to the senses, then the senses are to be trusted rather than reason. Many things are known by the senses to be so, yet the reasons for them remain unknown. Politely assuming that many of his antagonists have not properly understood what he said in De motu cordis, Harvey then recapitulates its contents with certain variations in detail. A few points here are of interest.

Although Harvey was in no doubt that the heart's movement as contractile muscle was the efficient cause of the circulation, here he seems to envisage its initiation in accordance with ancient belief rather than his own observation. The blood in its reservoir, especially the vena cava, when it arrives at the auricle swells and rises like leaven because of its own innate heat. It is this which causes the dilatation of the auricle which subsequently contracts through its own pulsific power and drives the blood into the right ventricle. This view, as will be seen later, derives from his studies of animal generation, as do also those which he expresses a little further on concerning the heart.[23] At this time, the publication of De generatione was much in his mind and it is not surprising to find that here he lays emphasis on the rôle of the blood, for he is thinking of the initiation of the circulation in the embryo rather than of its maintenance in the adult body. Accordingly he here denies to the heart some of the attributes with which it had been credited by common opinion, for he regards the blood, as he always had, as the primary vehicle of life. Saying that before long he hopes to publish abroad things that are still more wonderful and throw still greater light on natural philosophy, he continues:

> Yet in the mean time I will say and propound it without demonstration
> . . . that the heart, as it is the beginning of all things in the body, the
> spring, fountain, and first causer of life, is so to be taken, as being
> joyn'd together with the veins, and all the arteries, and the blood which
> is contained in them. . . . But if you understand by this word heart, the
> body of the heart, with the ventricles and ears, I do not think it to be
> the framer of the blood, and that it has not force, vertue, motion, or
> heat, as the gift of the heart (pp. 186–7).

Systole and diastole have different causes, and diastole always precedes
systole and is caused by innate heat:

> I think the first cause of distension is innate heat in the blood it self,
> which (like leaven) by little and little attenuated and swelling, is the last
> thing that is extinct in the creature. I agree to *Aristotle's* instance of
> pottage, or milk, in so far as he thinks that elevation, or depression of the
> blood, does not come of vapours, or exhalations, or Spirits rais'd into a
> vaporous or aereal form, nor is caus'd by any external agent, but by the
> regulating of Nature, an internal principle (p. 187).

So Harvey's opinion on the obscure motion of the blood ties up with
his observations of the punctum saliens in the embryo and with his
views on the nature of spirit as an integral part of the blood and its
vivifying force. Passing on to a discussion of the heat of the heart,
Harvey expresses the view that it does not resemble a charcoal fire or
a hot kettle,[24] nor is it the source of the heat of the blood. Rather it is
the blood which gives heat to the heart as is proved by the existence
of the coronary veins and arteries. It is this innate heat which is the
common instrument of every function and the prime cause of the pulse.
'This as yet I do not constantly aver, but propound it as a *Thesis*.'[25]
With a request that others will take up and discuss this hypothesis,
Harvey leaves the subject.

After a brief recapitulatory statement of the circulation which includes
the remarks that the blood passes from the arteries through the inter-
stices of the tissues into the veins, Harvey quotes another experiment
with an arm ligated for venesection to prove the return of blood through
the veins, and not through any anastomoses. If, when the veins have
swollen below the ligature, the whole arm be plunged into cold water
until it is chilled and then the bandage be suddenly released, the blood
will return with such speed to the heart that the subject may faint.
The swelling in the veins below the ligature cannot be caused by the
heat or ebullition of the blood, the cold water precludes it, but only by

the accumulation of the blood which cannot escape from the veins back into the arteries. And that blood does percolate through the tissues of the body is to be seen from those who have been hanged in whom all the parts beyond the noose, that is in the head, are engorged with blood, swollen and deep red in colour. If the noose be released, then in whatever position the body may be, in a short while the blood will leave these upper parts and percolate through the pores of the flesh to the lower parts which will become tumid and dark in colour. And if this happens in a body at the beginning of rigor, how much more easily must it happen in the living when the blood is not congealing and the pores are open and not compressed by the chill of death.

Finally, Harvey criticises Descartes's observations on the movement of the excised heart, pointing out that he is mistaken in what he believes to be diastole and what systole. The ventricles of the heart are only in diastole when they are filled with the blood driven into them by the auricles. Systole and diastole are contrary movements and have different causes. Descartes is wrong in believing with Aristotle that the cause of both is the ebullition in the blood.

> For these motions [sc. systole and diastole] are sudden strokes, and swift hits. And there is nothing that swells so . . ., or boyls up so suddenly, in the twinkling of an eye, and falls again; but [leaven] rises leisurely and falls suddenly: besides, in dissection you may by your own eyesight discern, that the ventricles of the heart are distended, and fill'd by the constriction of the ears, and are encreas'd in bignesse according as they are fill'd more or less, and that the distention of the heart, is a kind of violent motion, done by impulsion, not by an attraction (p. 191).

Harvey concludes the Letter with a list of 'dangerous sorts of diseases' which can follow from any accident happening to the circulation and the remarks that one day he hopes to publish all these things in a book of medical and pathological observations. Added as a tail-piece is the account of the experiment to prove the existence of the portal circulation and designed for Riolan's benefit.

While this Second Letter to Riolan is in some ways an appendix to *De motu cordis*, it is also important to realise that it is informed by Harvey's work on animal generation to a far greater extent than is the earlier book. At first sight, it may well be that certain views, notably on the heart, appear to contradict what he had said in *De motu cordis*, but when both these works are seen against the background of *De generatione* a clearer appreciation of what Harvey is trying to say can be had, and the persistent dilemma or antithesis in his thinking becomes apparent.

NOTES

1. In that year he is described as *Conseiller du Roi* on the title-page of the French edition of his anatomical works.
2. *Calendar of State Papers, Domestic, 1631–3*, p. 134.
3. Paris, Faculté de Médicine, MS. *Commentaires*, t. XII, 1622–36, ff.269ᵛ–276.
4. His assistants were François Vautour and Louis Henri Darquis.
5. André du Chemin died of apoplexy in Brussels on 27 October 1633 while in attendance on the Queen. His obituary notice describes him as a man of great piety and consummate erudition, 'fat and obese and of short stature, but worthy of a longer life'.
6. Riolan was 28 at the time, the same age as Vesalius when the *Fabrica* was written. But this book, Riolan explains, was too prolix and obscure to be understood by ignorant anatomists. His own work was designed to be a short, easy handbook for use by the students of medicine in Paris, both in public anatomies and in private dissections. It was not his first publication. As early as 1602, he was associated with his father in the production of a book in defence of the Faculté against the attacks of 'unorthodox', that is alchemical or Paracelsian, medicine. His first medical writings appeared in 1605. One, *Comparatio veteris medicinae cum nova*, is a general defence of orthodox or Hippocratic medicine, the other, *De monstro nato Lutetiae*, is an account of Siamese twins in which he shows himself more interested in the philosophical problems, such as whether they had one or two souls, than in the anatomical findings.
7. It is commonly said that Riolan was Dean of the Faculty of Medicine in Paris, but this was not the case. He did not at any time during his life hold that office. The mistake has arisen from the misunderstanding of the double meaning of the word *decanus* or *doyen*. Riolan is first so described in 1648 when Jacques Perreau was holding the office called by this name. In Riolan's case it simply means one of the most senior professors. In that year only two members of the Faculty were older than he and in 1649 he was the oldest and is called as well as *decanus*, 'antiquior magister'.
8. Riolan says of it that it is an abridgement of his *Anthropographia*, put out in small format to be convenient for students to carry around and know what he is talking about in his lessons and demonstrations, and also to remind him what he must show them for he believes in teaching anatomy by demonstration: 'I assure you, I do not seek to accommodate things to my opinion, but to submit my opinion to the nature of things, never believing that things that I had thought about in anatomy were necessarily so, until I had seen them many times and confirmed them by many investigations into different bodies. For this reason I write of and subscribe to only those things which I have seen.'

9. The similarity of Riolan's opinion with that of Descartes is evident: the continuing pulsation of the heart depends on the arrival of fresh blood, and this blood enters the heart drop by drop.

10. Harvey does not seem to make any mention of the time taken by the blood in making a complete circuit.

11. Harvey is less fair to Riolan when he accuses him of being unwilling to contradict what he had previously written in the *Anthropographia*. This very criticism Riolan anticipates in the prefatory letter to the *Encheiridium*, saying that second thoughts are often better than first and that differences between his works are to be explained by this.

12. Harvey's idea that the muscles assist the movement of the blood is not one that had just occurred to him. When speaking of the uses of the diaphragm in the *Prelectiones*, he gives as its fourth use: 'NB. WH perhaps it drives the blood and spirit to the guts and the limbs' (p. 245).

13. This Harvey did not do, but he discusses the lacteals in the letter which he wrote to Dr Robert Morison in 1652. See below, p. 207.

14. 'Therefore it is clear . . . what his opinion is, both of the Circulation of the blood through the whole bodie, as likewise through the lungs and the rest of the parts; for he that admits of the first Circulation, it is clear that he does not reject the other: For how can it be that he who has admitted of another Circulation through the whole body so often, and through the greater circulatory vessels, should deny that universal Circulation in any of the branches or parts of the second or third region? As if all the veins and those greater circulatory vessels, as he calls them, were not number'd by himself, and by all others, amongst the vessels of the second region. Is it possible that there should be a circulation through the whole body and not through the parts? and therefore where he denies it, he does it very stammeringly, and only staggers and palliates in his negations: there where he affirms, he speaks understandingly, and as becomes a Philosopher . . .' (p. 139).

15. 'Syringe' is the word used in the 1653 English text to translate the Latin *sipho*. ' . . . just as you might feel in the palm of your hand water squirted through a syringe at divers and severall shootings, so you may perceive, both by your sight and by its motion, the blood leaping out with a varying and unequall force. I have seen it sometimes in the cutting of the neck artery break out with such force, that the blood being forc'd against the hand, did by its reverberation and refraction, flye back four or five foot' (pp. 149–50). For the use of the analogy, see above, p. 170.

16. Willis, pp. 113–14, the 1653 English text is here imprecise and even incorrect.

17. See below, pp. 223–6.

18. The idea that the movement of the heart was the cause of its heat was held by Falloppius.

19. 'But it is manifest by our former experiment [*sc.* that with the bowls of arterial and venous blood], and by sense that the arterial blood is not so different, the influx of the blood and Spirit with it being not separate from the blood; but that it flows in one body through the arteries, sense may likewise make evident' (p. 161). When hands and feet are cold, it is the influx of blood which causes them to become warm again and return to their natural colour; in fact, when this blood returns too quickly they become engorged and painful from its too swift return

and over-great quantity. This fact Harvey had already observed in *De motu cordis*, cap. 11, and *De motu locali animalium*, p. 95: 'when spirit returns to a leg an excessive flow of blood ensues.'

20. See above, Conring's experiment, p. 160.
21. Willis, p. 122.
22. See above, p. 39. Sir Robert Darcy had suffered from an oppressive pain in the chest especially at night, so that he feared sometimes to die from syncope and sometimes from a paroxysmal suffocation and 'led an unquiet and anxious life.' He took many remedies on the advice of the College of Physicians, but in vain. The disease grew worse and he became dropsical and much distressed and finally died in one of his paroxysms. His body was opened in the presence of Dr Argent, then President of the College of Physicians (1625–8, 1629–34), and it was found that 'by the hinderance of the passage of the blood out of the left ventricle into the arteries, the wall of the left ventricle it self (which is seen to be thick and strong enough) was broken, and poured forth blood at a wide hole, for it was a hole so big, that it would easily receive one of my fingers' (p. 172). This is presumably one of the first descriptions of cardiac infarction.
23. See below, pp. 233–4.
24. Columbus had denied. that the heat of the heart in any way resembled a smouldering fire. See above, p. 50.
25. That is, a proposition to be maintained in a disputation.

Chapter Nine

The Last Letters 1651–1657

HARVEY's discovery of the circulation of the blood was a discovery made by a man at the height of his maturity. If, as has been suggested, the formulation of the hypothesis first occurred to him sometime between 1619 and 1625, then it was between the ages of 41 and 47. He published it complete with all the necessary experimental proofs when he was 50. His debate with Hofmann took place when he was 58 and his Letters to Riolan were not published until he was 71. During these years, Harvey was not at liberty to devote himself exclusively to the advancing of his own work in a laboratory; he was a busy physician with a practice in London and obligations to fulfil about the person of the King. He was deeply concerned with the business of the College of Physicians; he was sent on journeys with the Duke of Lennox, with the Earl of Arundel, journeys which removed him from England, and three times he attended King Charles on his visits to Scotland. When the Civil War broke out he was often absent from London in attendance on the King; he was present at the battle of Edgehill, and in December 1642 went with the Court to Oxford. There, in January 1645, he was made Warden of Merton College, and, as far as we know, there he stayed until the King left the city in April 1646. In November of that year he was with Charles at Newcastle. After that we lose sight of his movements and it is probable that from then on he was living retired, either in the house of his brother Eliab at Roehampton, or in that of his nephew Daniel at Coombe, near Croydon. Though he was a notorious Royalist he was not actively molested by the Parliamentary authorities. It was in the early part of the Civil War, while he was in attendance on the King, that his lodgings in Whitehall were plundered and, according to John Aubrey, he lost all his notes on the dissections of animals of different kinds together with the 'curious observations' he had made concerning them and the manuscript of the book he had written on insects.[1] That the action was deliberate and not accidental is plain from Harvey's account of it in *De generatione*:

> while I did attend upon his most Serene Majesty in these late distractions and more than Civil Wars, not only by the Parliament's permission but by its command, some rapacious hands spoiled me of all the goods in my house and (which I most lament) my adversaries stole from my study the notes which cost me many years industry (p. 418).

But Harvey was not, in 1643, assessed by the Parliamentary government for a forced loan as were his brothers Eliab and Daniel because of their Royalist sympathies. (When Daniel refused to pay, he was committed to prison and his estate seized until the obligation had been discharged in full.) After the King's death, Harvey certainly came under the order, passed in 1650, against 'delinquents' and forbidding any such to live or come within twenty miles of the City of London. (It would seem, therefore, that Harvey cannot have been living at Coombe at the time.) On 25 April 1650, the Council of State and Admiralty gave him a pass allowing him to visit London for fourteen days to attend his former patient, the Dowager Lady Thynne, in her sickness. This pass was granted 'on her engagement that he shall do nothing prejudicial to the commonwealth'. When the fourteen days were ended, on 6 May, a further licence was given him to remain in London for four more weeks, if the Lady Thynne were to live so long.[2] That these were unhappy years for Harvey there can be no doubt. He expresses his state of mind clearly enough in the reply he gave to George Ent's question 'Are all Affaires well, and right?'

> How can they be, he gravely answered, when the Commonwealth is surrounded with intestine troubles, and I myself as yet far from land, tossed in that tempestuous ocean? And unfeignedly, he added, if the comfort of my studies and the remembrance of many things long since fallen under my observation were not some refreshment to my mind, I know not what could prevail upon me to desire to survive the present.[3]

Harvey made no secret of his views, for he told Sir Charles Scarburgh that he had intended to endow a professorship of experimental philosophy at Cambridge and provide the university with a laboratory and a physic garden, had he not thought that by so doing he would be lending support to the religious and political opinions of the Commonwealth which he so much disliked.

> The University lost, as we have said, this most splendid Institute, projected by our Harvey, robbed by the inequity of those most wicked times. I see, he said (for he often spoke to me of this matter and not without tears in his eyes and mine), I see plainly that, were I to dedicate my fortune, as I had intended, to the promoting of the knowledge of truth and to the public weal, I should do nothing other than make Anabaptists, Fanatics and all manner of thieves and parricides my heirs.[4]

By 1650 the storm which the publication of *De motu cordis* had provoked was over, and the younger generation at least were convinced of the truth of Harvey's hypothesis. But Riolan still remained obdurate. In 1649 he published a volume of *Opuscula anatomica nova* in which he speaks of the renewing of medicine by means of the new doctrine of the circulatory movement of the blood (Instauratio magna Physicae et medicinae per novam doctrinam de motu circulatorio sanguinis in corde), and attacks two letters of Walaeus written in defence of the Harveyan circulation. It is to this work that Harvey alludes in the First Letter saying that he had not then seen it.[5] It was followed in 1652 by the publication of Riolan's own *Tractatus de motu sanguinis eiusque circulatione vera ex doctrina Hippocratis*, and by his reply to Harvey's Letters: *Responsio ad duas exercitationes anatomicas postremas Guillelmi Harvei Angli*. In all these and in other publications in 1653 and 1655, Riolan continued to reiterate his own peculiar theory of the circulation. Meantime, in 1650, Paul Marquard Slegel[6] had joined issue with Riolan in a book published from Hamburg entitled *De sanguinis motu commentatio in qua praecipue in Joannis Riolani sententiam inquiritur*. In it Slegel attacks Riolan's preposterous notion of different circulations and in particular criticises what he had said concerning the function of the portal vein. For many years Slegel had been a supporter of Harvey and had even attempted, in 1638, to convince Caspar Hofmann of the truth of the circulation, but to no effect.[7] His attempts to convince Riolan were likewise futile. On 26 March 1651, Harvey wrote to Slegel to thank him for a copy of this book. He had himself intended to write against Riolan's most recent arguments, but as he had been very busy with the publication of *De generatione*, had had no time, and was therefore delighted that Slegel should have so skilfully refuted all Riolan's attacks on the circulation and overthrown his latest opinions. He then

203

refers to Riolan's persistent refusal to allow the passage of the blood from the right to the left ventricle of the heart by way of the lungs and his continuing belief in the existence of pores in the septum of the heart.

In this belief, Riolan was not alone. In 1635, the French philosopher and mathematician Pierre Gassendi had published a small treatise *De septo cordis pervio observatio* in which he described how he had seen at an anatomy at Aix, one of the professors of anatomy, a surgeon named Payanus, demonstrate a hole through the septum. 'He did not try to push the instrument straight through, but first introducing the tip . . . pushed onwards very gently, twisting the probe upwards and downwards and from side to side most patiently . . . until at last it penetrated into the left ventricle.' Accused of making the hole, he requested one of those present to cut through the septum down to his probe and when this was done a small winding passage lined with a thin and glistening membrane was seen. Gassendi reasonably concludes that, as the passage exists, it must have a use, and this use is to allow the more subtle portion of the blood to be sucked through into the left ventricle, and it either percolates drop by drop, as is the general opinion, or abundantly as seems to be Harvey's opinion. In spite of the fact that Gassendi had supported Harvey's theory of the circulation throughout the body, he seems to have had no idea that Harvey utterly denied any passage through the septum of the heart.

The experiment to prove incontrovertibly that there are no porosities in the interventricular septum Harvey describes at the beginning of his letter to Slegel. He says that he had recently performed it in the presence of several of his colleagues. It is the last of all his experiments in connection with the circulation and like all the earlier ones is of masterly simplicity. Harvey himself describes it as ἄφυκτον, that is, one which cannot be set aside, yet in his own view it was unnecessary for the existence of the circulation implied that no such pores existed. Having tied the pulmonary artery, pulmonary veins and aorta in a cadaver and made an incision into the left ventricle of the heart, he inserted a tube through the vena cava into the right ventricle and through this tube forcibly injected the greater part of a pound of warm water. The result was that the right auricle and ventricle were enormously distended but not one single drop of water or blood made its escape through the hole in the left ventricle. He then untied the ligatures and inserted the tube into the pulmonary artery which was tightly ligated between the point of insertion and the heart so that no water could go back into the right ventricle. When the water was forced into the pulmonary artery towards the lungs, immediately a torrent of water mixed with blood escaped through the hole in the left ventricle. The amount that escaped through this hole was equal in quantity to the amount that was injected. 'You may try this experiment as often as you please, and you will always find it thus.' This one experiment, Harvey concludes, will put an end to all Riolan's theories which are utterly without any experimental foundation. Riolan, says Harvey, has been playing the advocate and not acting like a practised anatomist and, as Aristotle says, you cannot expect an advocate to demonstrate his proof.

Harvey goes on to discuss the question of anastomoses between veins and arteries, saying that he wishes he had been more precise in what he had written about them in his Letters to Riolan. Because he was there arguing against Riolan's view that the circulation was confined to the larger vessels only, he was led to assert that there were no anastomoses in the Galenic sense. 'I have never found any visible anastomoses.' He had, however, also admitted that he had found their equivalent in three places, in the plexus of the brain, in the spermatic veins and arteries and in the umbilical veins and arteries. The intercommunication of veins and arteries by means of osculations, which was the Galenic opinion and the one commonly held in Harvey's time, he utterly denies. The belief in the existence of anastomoses of this kind was linked with the idea that the blood ebbed and flowed in the veins and arteries, and moreover, that it ebbed and flowed indiscriminately from the veins to the arteries and from the arteries to the veins. The circulation of the blood proves that there is both an out-going and an in-flowing of blood, but also that it occurs in different places and at different times and in different sets of vessels. The blood is transferred from the veins to the arteries only through the medium of the heart whose valves are contrived to that purpose. Harvey had, therefore, assumed that it was by some other 'admirable artifice' that the transference from the arteries to the veins was effected, at least wherever there was no direct transudation through the flesh. For this reason, and also because he had never been able to find them, he doubted the truth of the whole of the ancient notions concerning anastomoses. He finds further support for this rejection in the fact that he has seen something equivalent to these anastomoses in the three places he has named where the blood is transferred from the arteries to the veins and where there is a mechanism to prevent the regurgitation of the blood delivered into the veins back into the arteries.

He explains this mechanism by analogy with the conjunction which is to be found between the ureters and the bladder, the bile duct and the duodenum. The arteries in their ultimate ramifications are much smaller than the veins they accompany and which they approach more and more closely until they are lost inside the coats of the veins. So the ureters insinuate themselves obliquely into the coats of the bladder, without anything in the nature of an osculatory anastomosis. It is quite easy if you try to fill the bladder with air or water through the ureters, but impossible to drive this air or water back from the bladder into the ureters. The transference of the blood from the arteries to the veins does not happen through anastomoses in the ancient meaning of the word, because this implies a free passage for the blood in both directions and this does not happen. Once the blood has got into the vein, it cannot go back into the artery from which it came. And the right explanation of this phenomenon is not, as Slegel had suggested, anything to do with the impulse of the blood through the arteries. To prove this, tie the aorta near the left ventricle in a living animal and drain all the blood from the arteries. It will then be seen that the veins are still full of blood which proves that the blood does not move back spontaneously into the arteries, nor can it be driven back by force. The blood is driven into the veins by the impulse given to it in the arteries; it is not drawn into them after the manner in which air is drawn into bellows when they expand. The explanation of the findings in the experiment just mentioned of ligating the aorta is furnished by analogy with the ureters and the bladder. Another reason why anastomoses in the ancient sense cannot exist, is that as the arteries are always much smaller than the veins which they approach, their sides cannot conjoin in such a way as to form a common meatus, for things which join in this way must be of equal size. If there were anastomoses between them, the veins and arteries would not go, as they do, straight to the extremities of the body where their tips meet. Moreover, if they were conjoined by mutual inosculations, the veins would also pulsate like the arteries by reason of the continuity of the parts.

Harvey's wishes that Slegel would continue with the work that he was doing were not fulfilled. He died in Hamburg in 1653. Riolan was still not convinced and, as has already been said, continued to publish his own mistaken opinions on the circulation. Harvey's last word on Riolan was written in his letter to John Daniel Horst of Hesse-Darmstadt on 1 February 1655:

With regard to the views of Riolan and his opinion on the circulation of the blood, it is quite obvious that he is making a great effort to produce great nonsense; nor do I see that he has as yet satisfied anyone with his figments. Slegel wrote more accurately and more modestly, and, had the fates allowed, would undoubtedly have taken the edge off his arguments and his abuse too. But Slegel, as I learn and grieve to learn, laid aside this mortal life some months ago.

The last remarks which Harvey made on the subject of the circulation relate to the action of the heart. They occur in the letter which he wrote on 28 April 1652 to Dr Robert Morison of Paris.[8]

The heart rejoices in three kinds of motion, namely the systole in which the heart contracts itself and expels the blood contained within it, and next a kind of relaxation, a movement which is the opposite of the former one and in which the fibres of the heart appropriated to motion are slackened. These two motions inhere in the very substance of the heart, just as they do in all other muscles. The remaining motion is diastole in which the heart is distended by the blood impelled from its auricles into its ventricles; and the ventricles replete and distended in this manner stimulate the heart to contract itself, and this motion always precedes the systole which will follow immediately afterwards.

This description is far removed from Harvey's avowed bewilderment on first watching a beating heart and to which he had confessed in *De motu cordis* saying: 'I was almost tempted to think . . . that the motion of the heart was only to be comprehended by God.'

This letter to Morison, however, is chiefly concerned with a discussion of the lymphatic system. The lacteal vessels had been discovered in 1622 by Gaspare Aselli, professor of anatomy at Padua, and their description published in 1627, after Aselli's death. In 1647, the French anatomist, Jean Pecquet, identified the thoracic duct and the *receptaculum chyli* and their termination in the left subclavian vein. His findings were published in 1651 in his *Experimenta nova anatomica*, and it was of this book that Morison had asked Harvey's opinion. In his letter, Harvey says that he had observed these 'white canals' even before Aselli's book was published, but he cannot agree with him in thinking that they carry chyle. He does not think that the fluid which they carry is different from milk and would wish to have it demonstrated by reason and experiment that it was in fact chyle. He thinks that the vessels are too small and too variable for this purpose. Moreover, chyle is not at all times and in all animals of the consistency and colour of milk but varies with the food eaten, as does the colour of the urine. Moreover, traces of it ought to be found in the intestines, for mere percolation through the coats of the intestines is too short a process to allow the fluid to change its nature and assume the appearance of milk. He disagrees with Pecquet in thinking that the motion of this 'milky fluid' has anything to do with respiration, but if chyle were transported from the intestines to the subclavian veins, then it would have to be admitted that, before reaching the heart, the chyle mixed with the blood which was about to enter the right auricle and ventricle. But why should it not be supposed that the chyle enters directly into the mesenteric veins and there mixes with the blood, thus being perfected by the heat and serving for the nutrition of the parts?

> For the heart itself can be esteemed of greater importance than the other parts, or called the fountain of heat and life, for no other reason than that it contains within itself a larger quantity of blood, and this blood, as Aristotle said, is not contained in veins as it is in the other parts, but in an ample cavity and, as it were, a cistern.

Confirmation of this opinion Harvey finds in the great number of arteries and veins distributed to the intestines and in his knowledge that embryos are nourished by means of the umbilical vessels by the circulating blood. He does not see why the manner of nourishment should be different in the adult. From this opinion Harvey did not deviate, in spite of several letters to him from those directly concerned in attempting to elucidate the use of the lacteals, and he continued to demand proof that the vessels actually contained chyle. Finally, in 1655, in a letter to John Daniel Horst, he excused himself from any further part in the debate saying that age and illness had destroyed any wish to 'explore new subtleties, and after long labours my mind is too fond of peace and quiet to let myself become too deeply involved in an arduous discussion on recent discoveries. So I am far from setting myself up as a suitable mediator in this dispute.'[9] To this weariness he gave final expression in the letter he wrote a few weeks before his death to Dr Jon Vlackfeld of Haarlem: 'It is useless for you to spur me on to gird myself to any new investigation seeing that I am now not only ripe in years but also weary. It seems to me, indeed, that I am entitled to ask for my honorable discharge from duty.' On 3 June 1657, Harvey died.

NOTES

1. 'I remember I have heard him say he wrote a booke de insectis, which he had been many yeares about, & had made curious researches and antomicall observations on them; this booke was lost when his lodgings at Whitehall were plundered in the time of the Rebellion: he could never for love nor money retrive them or heare what became of them and sayed *'twas the greatest crucifying to him that ever he had in all his life.'* See Keynes, *Life*, p. 436.

2. *Calendar of State Papers, Domestic, 1650*, pp. 537, 540.

3. From the Epistle Dedicatory to Harvey's *Anatomical Exercitations concering . . . Generation*, London 1653, sig. A.3ᵛ.

4. From Sir Charles Scarburgh's Harveian Oration, Oxford, Bodleian Library, MS Rawlinson D 815, f. 6ᵛ.

5. It was registered in the Stationers' Register in London, 25 June 1649.

6. Slegel was born in 1605, the son of a prosperous merchant of Hamburg. He studied medicine in Altdorf and by 1628 was working with Rolfinck in Wittenberg. In 1631 he started on a journey through Europe and visited France, where he met Riolan in Paris, Holland, and probably England where he may have met Harvey. He then went to Italy and signed the matriculation register of the German Nation in the University of Padua on 20 October 1635. He was promoted doctor of medicine and philosophy of that university in 1637. In 1638 he became professor of medicine in Jena with the obligation to teach botany, anatomy and surgery. From August 1640 until February 1641 he was Rector of the University of Jena. About this time he became physician to the Dukes of Saxony and on 11 October 1642 he left Jena to become official physician to the city of Hamburg where he died in 1653. See *Geschichte der Universität Jena, 1548/58–1958*, Jena 1958, vol. I, p. 148; and on his debate with Riolan, K. E. Rothschuh, 'Jean Riolan jun. (1580–1657) in Streit mit Paul Marquart Schlegel (1605–1653) am die Blutbewegungslehre Harveys', *Gesnerus*, XXI (1964), 72–82.

7. 'Though my ever greatly valued teacher Hofmann taught me and others the first beginnings of the circulation from the structure and use of the heart and lungs, whence it became easy to understand the new movement of the blood, yet he himself could never be brought to admit the circular course of the blood. Even Harvey could not prevail so far, either in person, when he visited Hofmann during his German journey, or by letters which he several times sent to him; nor did I succeed in obtaining his consent in many discussions with him in 1638, when I was welcomed in his house, where I stayed for four months.' From the Preface to his *De sanguinis motu commentatio*, quoted by Keynes, *Life*, p. 237.

8. Dr Robert Morison (1620–83) studied first in the University of Aberdeen where he became a doctor of philosophy in 1638. After fighting in the Civil War on the King's side he went to Paris where he studied science, and in 1648 became a doctor of medicine of the University of Angers. In the following year he became physician to Gaston, duke of Orleans. He returned to England at the Restoration and became senior physician and king's botanist to Charles II. In 1669 he was made professor of botany in the University of Oxford, where he remained until his death. He wrote various botanical works and is known as a taxonomist. The genus *Morisonia* perpetuates his name.

Chapter Ten

De Generatione Animalium *and the Final Assessment*

THE last published work of Harvey, his *Exercitationes de generatione animalium*, was printed in London in March 1651. The story of how Dr George Ent visited him in his retirement and succeeded in carrying off the manuscript is well known.

> Having returned him very many thanks for so high a favour, I took my leave and departed like another Jason enriched with the Golden Fleece. And when upon my return home, I had surveyed the book, I could not but wonder that so vast a treasure had lain so long concealed.[1]

This visit probably took place 'about Christmas' in 1648,[2] so that the final draft of the book was probably completed sometime between 1647 and 1648 at the latest, that is, before the publication of the Letters to Riolan, though perhaps not before the writing of the Second Letter. A suspicion that it may have been written even earlier seems confirmed by the evidence which has recently been discovered that at least a draft of it, or some part of the manuscript, was seen in 1638 by Sir Thomas Browne.[3] The book had indeed remained long concealed for Harvey had been collecting material for it throughout the whole of his life and possibly writing and emending different sections at different times. 'The examination of the bodies of animals has always been my delight', Harvey said to Ent when he visited him, and in this book he recalls how, once, in Padua, in the spring season at the beginning of the century, he had helped Fabricius and had himself made observations on a cock and two hens 'that I might have some knowledge of the time during which coition is most successful and the necessity therefore' (p. 19). That by

1616 the work was already well under way is proved by the number of observations which occur in the Anatomical Lectures and which are repeated in this book. It has been suggested that Harvey's investigations of the King's deer took place between 1630 and 1635,[4] but he himself seems to imply a longer period than this, for he speaks of the 'long series of years' (p. 218) during which he had observed the process of generation in the hind and doe. He explains how he had had the opportunity to dissect numbers of these animals as often as he wanted, for, since he came to man's estate, King Charles had been in the habit of hunting almost every week, the buck in the summer months and the doe in the autumn and winter, 'no Prince in the world having greater store of deer' (p. 217). A number of the observations on deer occurring in this book had already been made by 1616. As late as his stay in Oxford, 1642–46, Harvey was still investigating the development of the chick embryo, for John Aubrey records that he did daily examine hen's eggs that were hatching in Dr George Bathurst's rooms in Trinity, 'to discerne the progres and way of Generation'.[5] As no complete investigation of the text of Harvey's *De generatione* has as yet been undertaken, it is impossible in our present state of knowledge to disentangle the various layers of its composition, to decide what was first written and what last. It can only be taken as a whole and as such considered as the background to Harvey's whole work, a source to which we can turn for illumination of ideas adumbrated in his other writings but not there discussed in any detail as being irrelevant to the matter in hand. As such it is of capital importance in the understanding of Harvey's work, and this apart from its own peculiar importance as one of the first major works in embryology.

The reason which Harvey gives to Ent for having delayed the publication of this book, was his wish to avoid the occurrence of a storm similar to that which the publication of *De motu cordis* had provoked.

> You know full well what great troubles my former lucubrations raised. Better is it certainly at some times to grow wise at home, than by the hasty divulgation of such things, to the knowledge whereof you have attained with vast labour, to stir up tempests that may deprive you of your leisure and your quiet for the future (pp. a2–a2ᵛ).

The novelty in this work was Harvey's view that epigenesis and not pre-formation explained the order of the development of the parts in the embryo, and he may well have feared that this view would provoke a storm, for although it was Aristotelian in origin it was contrary to the current belief. It may also be that he thought the work incomplete, not only because he had lost all his notes on the generation of insects and much besides, but because he could bring it to no definite conclusion in the same way that he had brought *De motu cordis*. It was not a subject which, without a microscope, was capable of experimental proof, and he is forced to end with an hypothesis and a plea for its acceptance, or at least for its serious consideration.

It has sometimes been said that *De generatione* lacks form and order and is little better than a shapeless collection of notes. But this is not the case. While it is true that it is discursive and to a certain extent repetitive, it has, nevertheless, a plan. In the Introduction, Harvey explains that there are three main topics to be discussed: first, the order of generation of the parts in the embryo and the foetus; second, the primary matter out of which generation is made and its efficient cause; third, the faculties of the formative and vegetative 'soul' deduced from its works, and the nature of the soul from its organs and their functions. These topics are built into the structure of the book as is evident from an analysis of its chapters. Of its total of seventy-two, the first twenty-five chapters are concerned with the anatomy of the hen's uterus,[6] the formation of the egg in the uterus, successive examinations of hatching eggs from the first to the seventh day, on the fourteenth day and at birth, and the various deductions that can be made from these observations. This section has its parallel from the sixty-third to the seventieth chapter where Harvey considers the generation of viviparous animals as exemplified by the hind and doe, and based on examinations of the gravid uterus of hinds made at monthly intervals from September to December. Between these two sections fall three others, in the first of which (caps 26–41) he considers the part played respectively by the hen and the cock in the generation of the egg in utero, and in the third (caps 58–61) the nutrition of the chick in the egg and the uses of the various parts of the egg. The central section of the book (caps 43–57) considers how the chick grows in the egg, the substance of which it is formed, the causes of its generation and the order in which the parts appear. Into this also comes incidentally the consideration of the nature of the formative and vegetative 'soul'. The last two chapters of the book pick up and discuss further the problems of innate heat and primigenial moisture, both of which appear in the central section. At the end of the book are three short treatises which do not seem to be an integral part of it, but are more in the nature of appendices and may well not have been composed at the same time as the main part of the book. The first, on Parturition, reveals Harvey's considerable knowledge of obstetrics and gynaecology. The second, on the uterine membranes and humours, is largely a criticism of Fabricius's work and is filled with anatomical observations on a diversity of creatures. It contains his conclusion that the placenta is analogous to the liver and re-emphasises his statements that the circulation in the foetus is distinct from that of the mother and that the life of the one is separate from that of the other. The third, on conception, reiterates Harvey's views on the manner in which this is achieved. It is, perhaps, the most obviously Aristotelian of all his writings.

The main problems which Harvey seeks to investigate in this book are then, how conception is effected, what is the part of the male and what of the female, how heredity is explained, how life is transmitted, and what this living thing is, in what order the parts appear in the embryo and in the foetus and how they are nourished. Without a microscope and consequently no knowledge of microscopical anatomy, with a very limited knowledge of physiology and none at all of bio-chemistry, these were problems which, for the most part, he could not hope to solve. His contributions to the subject were, therefore, confined to the observations which he could make with the naked eye or with a single lens. In the circumstances, their quality and accuracy is remarkable. How far he succeeded or failed in his purpose, how his work compares with that of his contemporaries, are problems with which we are not here concerned, any more than with a discussion of his ideas on generation as a whole. We will merely attempt to examine those parts of it which underlie his thinking on the movement of the heart and blood, and consequently limit the discussion to his views on the blood and on the heart, on spirits and soul, and on the purpose of the circulation.

Harvey's knowledge of the circulation of the blood informs the whole of the book. It is directly referred to on several occasions: 'I perceive that the wonderful Circulation of the Blood, first found out by me, is consented to by almost all, and that no man hath hitherto made any objection to it greatly worth a confutation'[7] (p. 154); 'And lastly, from the constitution of the umbilical vessels in the egg . . . we may collect a circular movement of the blood (such as we have long since demonstrated in our little book *De motu sanguinis in animalibus*) . . .

213

(p. 166). Harvey's continuing observations on animals were still adding to the subject of the circulation, but *De generatione* contains only one piece of experimental evidence not recorded in *De motu cordis*. It was collected after 1626 and is alluded to in the Anatomical Lectures,[8] and is the fact that air blown into the ovarian arteries finds its way into the neighbouring veins, while the arteries cannot be inflated by air blown into the veins, and this 'is a prevalent argument for the Circulation of the Blood, which was my invention, for it doth clearly evince a passage from the arteries into the veins, but no retreat from the veins into the arteries again' (p. 222).

Though Harvey had observed the movement of the heart a thousand times in vivisections of a great diversity of animals, he had never watched the beating of a human heart until he saw it in the body of the eldest son of the Viscount Montgomery.[9] As a child he had had a severe fall which broke the ribs on his left side. The resulting wound did not heal, but left a large cavity through which it was thought the lungs could be seen. When news of this came to the ears of Charles I, he sent Harvey to see the boy. Harvey, finding that it was in fact the heart which was visible, brought the young man to Court that the King might see for himself and watch the movement of the heart and touch the ventricles as they contracted. So Harvey could confirm in a human subject that systole was indeed contraction, and the moment at which the heart rose up and struck the chest wall, and that the systole of the heart coincided with the diastole of the arteries.

> We likewise took notice of the movement of his heart, namely, that in its diastole it was drawn in and retracted, and in its systole came forth and was thrust out, and that the systole was made in the heart at the moment when the diastole was perceptible in the wrist; that the proper motion and function of the heart was its systole; and lastly, that the heart beats upon the breast and is a little prominent when it is lifted upwards and contracted into itself (p. 157).

It is of some interest to notice that in his Anatomical Lectures (p. 233), Harvey had given a complete reference to Galen's statement that he had seen the movement of the heart in a boy whose sternum was 'perforated'. This was the slave of Maryllus the mime-writer, and he had suffered a blow on the sternum in the wrestling school. As a result of neglect, suppuration of the sternum ensued and Galen excised the bone leaving the heart visible. As the reference to this does not occur in

Bauhin's textbook which Harvey was so closely following for his Lectures, it is obvious that Harvey's own particular interest in the occurrence led to the inclusion of the quotation.[10]

In *De motu cordis*, cap. 16, Harvey makes a direct reference to his work on animal generation. In between a sketch of the portal circulation and a description of the content of the splenic branch of the portal vein, he digresses on to the subject of the liver and to the fact that it plays no part in the circulation in the foetus. His observations have shown him that in the first forming of the foetus, the liver is made last. He then discusses the umbilical vessels of the embryo in the egg, points out that the chick is first nourished by the white part and subsequently by the yolk which can still be found in its belly several days after its hatching.

> But we shall speak of these things more conveniently in our observations concerning the forming of births [*sc.* foetuses], where there may be many enquiries of this nature, why this is first made and perfected, and that afterwards; and of the principalitie of Members, what part is the cause of another; and many things likewise concerning the heart, As why (as *Aristotle, de partibus Animalium 3*) it was made the first consistent and seems to have in it life, motion, and sense, before any thing of the rest of the body be perfected: And likewise of the blood, why before all things and how it has in it the beginning of life and of the creature: why it requires to be mov'd and driven up and down; and then for what cause the heart seems to have been made (p. 100).

It is clear from this quotation that Harvey saw no inherent contradiction between the statement that the heart has life, motion and sensation before all the rest of the body, and that the blood is the beginning of the life of the creature and the heart the instrument that effects its movement. The first statement is Aristotelian; the second derives from Harvey's embryological observations. That he believed both in the 'primacy of the Heart' and the 'antiquity of the blood', as these notions have been called, from at least 1616 is evident from various statements made in the Anatomical Lectures. It could be maintained that when he is referring to the primacy of the heart in the Lectures he is doing so because he is quoting Aristotle. Statements such as 'all things are connected with the heart, wherefore it has pride of place and is the essential first principle of a man just as the centre is of a circle' (p. 29), and 'the chest, the abode of the heart, the inner room, the shrine, where is the fount of heat, the vital spirits, emotion, the passions and respiration' (p. 33), and again 'According to Aristotle, the heart is the primary organ

215

of all living creatures and consequently the place where the blood is made' (p. 125); all these are in fact quotations from Aristotle's *De partibus animalium* and may or may not represent ideas with which he is in total agreement. That in his own mind, there is some limitation to be applied to Aristotle's views seems to follow from his saying of the heart: 'WH it is the chiefest of all the parts of the body not on its own account . . . but on account of the abundance of blood and spirit which exists in the ventricles, for which reason it is the source of all the heat in the body' (p. 249). Beside these quotations can be set others exemplifying his ideas on the antiquity of the blood: 'Blood is rather the author of the viscera than they of it, because blood is in being before the viscera' (p. 127); 'WH nor is the heart the chief part by virtue of its origin, for I think that the ventricles . . . are made from the drop of blood which is found in the egg, and the heart is fashioned along with the remaining parts, as sprouts come forth in an ear of corn, all together from something which is too small to be seen' (p. 251); and finally, a direct disagreement with Aristotle arising from his own embryological observations: 'Therefore Aristotle against the opinion of the doctors deemed that the primary source of blood was not in the liver but in the heart, because in the liver there is no blood outside the veins. WH rather it is blood which is the primary source of both the liver and the heart as I have seen' (p. 257). As will be seen, both sets of ideas are expressed in all Harvey's published works. Consequently, they must not be thought of as contradictory, but complementary, and the key to Harvey's own understanding of them is provided by the quotation already given from the Lectures in which he limits the Aristotelian notion of the heart's primacy and subscribes to it only because of the peculiar relation of the heart to the blood. This antithesis between the heart and the blood is fundamental to Harvey's thought. Sometimes it inclines more towards the primacy of the heart, as in *De motu cordis* where the central rôle of the heart is of paramount importance to the whole theory of the circulation of the blood, and sometimes, when thinking in more general terms, it inclines to stress the antiquity of the blood. That the full explanation of the two ideas and of their balance is to be found in *De generatione* will be seen from what follows.

From his observations on fecundated eggs,[11] Harvey formed the opinion that the embryo develops by epigenesis, an opinion which was not generally accepted until the nineteenth century. He found a similar process in the development of the foetus in the uterus of the hind,[12] and concluded that all animal generation was effected in a similar manner and that all creatures came from some kind of egg. His conclusions on the order of the generation of the parts are summed up in his short treatise 'On the uterine membranes and humours', where he says that first there is the primordium or rudiment, then in the hen's egg, the colliquament, and in the uterus a clear liquid enclosed in the amnion which is itself enclosed in the chorion. In this a red point appears and in due course pulsates and from it arise 'rays' of vessels. In the hen's egg, Harvey focussed his attention on what Fabricius had called the *cicatricula*, or 'little scar', a white and very small circle apparent in the investing membrane of the vitellus.

> This is a very little spot, about the bigness of a small lentil, like the pupil of a small bird's eye, and white, flat and round. ... it is ... the most important part of the whole egg for whose sake all the rest of the parts are created, the original and foundation out of which the chick itself is formed (p. 35).

On the second day of incubation this cicatricula is seen to have enlarged in size and to be divided into circles 'as they might be drawn with a pair of compasses, and having a very small white point for their centre' (p. 46). By the third day, the circles of the cicatricula have become the size of the nail of the ring-finger, or larger, and divide the spot clearly, and within them is a clear white fluid, the colliquament. In the very centre is a white speck. By the fourth day, the margin of the fluid has a reddish appearance,

> and in the centre almost of it, there leaps a capering bloody point, which is yet so exceeding small that in its dilation it flasheth like the smallest spark of fire, and presently upon its contraction quite escapes the eye and disappears (p. 49).

This red palpitating spot, the punctum saliens, is soon seen to consist of two parts, each of which reciprocates the movement of the other, 'in such order and manner that whilst one is contracting, the other is swollen with blood and shines ruddy in colour, the which being presently contracted discharges itself of the blood that was in it, and, a moment of time intervening the former swells again and repeats the pulse. And so you may easily see that the action of these vesicles is contraction by which the blood is driven and pumped into the vessels' (p. 53). Some such pulsating point as this in the uterus of a hind, Harvey showed the King on one November day:

it was then so small that, without the advantage of the sun's beams obliquely falling upon it, he could not have perceived its shivering motion (p. 232).

It was from these and observations like them that Harvey concluded that blood exists before the pulse, that it is the first part of the embryo which may be said to live, that from it the body of the embryo is made and from it also is derived the nourishment by which the embryo lives, 'and that it is, if anything be, the primary generative particle' (p. 59). From it are formed the blood vessels and the heart, and in due time the liver and the brain.

This is the same conclusion which Harvey had already reached in 1616, but whereas we do not know whether by this date he was completely satisfied that his observations were sufficient to validate his conclusion, by 1628 he was certainly convinced of their truth, for in *De motu cordis*, cap. 4, he says:

> In a Hen's egg I shewed the first beginning of the Chick, like a little cloud, by putting an egg off which the shell was taken, into water warm and clear, in the midst of which cloud there was a point of blood which did beat, so little, that when it was contracted it disappeared, and vanish'd out of our sight, and in its dilatation, shew'd itself again red and small, as the point of a needle; in so much as betwixt being seen and not being seen, as it were betwixt being and not being, it did represent a beating, and the beginning of life (p. 34).
>
> But if you observe the fashioning of a Chick in the egg, first of all there is in it as I said only a bladder or drop of blood, which beats, and encreasing afterwards the heart is perfected; so in some creatures (as not reaching a further perfection) there is a certain little bladder only like a point, red or white, as the beginning of life, as in Bees, Wasps, Snails, Shrimps, Crayfish (pp. 33–4).

In this chapter also, Harvey adds a refinement to these observations by noticing that from the blood, from this pulsating vesicle, the auricles of the heart are formed first and later the ventricles. He has been discussing the fact that the right auricle appears to be the last part of the heart to die, and that even after that there seems to be some kind of movement in the blood in the right auricle, and he continues:

> A thing of like nature, in the first generation of a living creature most evidently appears in a Hen's egg within seven dayes after her sitting; first of all there is in it a drop of blood, which moves, as *Aristotle* like-

wise observed, which receiving encrease, and the Chicken being form'd in part, the ears of the heart are fashioned, which beating there is always life; then afterwards within a few days the body beginning to receive its lineaments, then likewise is the body of the heart framed, but for some days it appears whitish and without blood, as the rest of the body, nor doth it beat and move (p. 31).

So that if a man will more narrowly pry into the truth, he will not say, that the heart is the first thing that lives, and the last that dies, but rather the ears, ... and that it both lives before the heart and dies after it (p. 32).

There can, therefore, be no doubt that whatever Harvey may say in *De motu cordis* about the primacy of the heart, and he says a great deal, he was quite certain that the blood was in existence before the heart and that the heart was formed from this blood. But in *De motu cordis* the heart is of prime importance. It is the action of the heart which drives the blood, and this is what his contemporaries did not believe and what Harvey is concerned to prove, and to prove moreover that the action of the heart drives the blood in a circle. Whether the blood exists in the embryo before the formation of the heart, what is the relationship of the heart to the blood, these are subjects which are irrelevant to the main theme of the book. As has already been seen,[13] he says that he will discuss them elsewhere.

Harvey first alludes to the purpose of the heart's action in his Anatomical Lectures where he quotes Aristotle's view that it is to no purpose but is a passive action like that which is seen in boiling pottage.[14] This he counters by pointing out that when the heart is wounded, it discharges blood and not air. Consequently the idea that it contains air is nonsense, and, by inference, so also is Aristotle's idea of ebullition in the heart. But that the action of the heart is for some purpose 'is shown by its construction, its fibres, valves and the artery itself.' He then proceeds to ask a series of questions which he does not answer:

> WH is it cooled by the boiling movement of the blood? or are the parts warmed by the arterial blood which would explain why when an artery is obstructed that piece of the body becomes cold? WH or is it to assist in the dissipating of heat in fevers and other morbid conditions engendered by heat? (p. 273)

This raises the problem of Harvey's views on innate heat. Aristotle had held that innate heat was the originator of everything in the body and that the heart was the source of this heat which it imparted to all the members. So in his Lectures, Harvey wrote:

> Wherefore seeing that the heart imparts heat to all the parts and receives it from none, it is the citadel and abode of heat, the presiding god of this edifice, the fountain and conduit-head (p. 251).

But these are not original remarks. They are common-places to the seventeenth-century way of thinking and they all ultimately derive from Aristotle. For the moment, however, Harvey is not concerned to decide whether innate heat originates in the heart, or whether it originates in the blood and is transmitted to the heart by the blood. He has observed that warmth is carried to the parts by the blood and that this blood is driven into the arteries by the heart which is a very strong muscle; somehow warmth is conveyed along with the blood. The conclusions which he reaches in *De motu cordis* on the use of the circulation are not far different. They occur in cap. 8, in a passage which he explains to Hofmann is merely a suggestion of what might be and is not to be taken as an authoritative statement of a fact. These conclusions derive from his notion of innate heat as the cherisher of life, and of the heart as a muscle which propels the blood warmed by the innate heat within it, throughout the whole body. The difference between this and the previous statement and the reason for which Harvey insists that this is only a tentative suggestion, is that here he has firmly situated innate heat in the body of the heart itself.

> So in all likelihood it comes to pass in the body, that all the parts are nourished, cherished, and quickened with blood, which is warm, perfect, vaporous, full of spirit, and, that I may say so, alimentative; in the parts the blood is refrigerated, coagulated, and made as it were barren; from thence it returns to the heart, as to the fountain or inmost shrine of the body, to recover its perfection, and there again by natural heat, powerful and vehement, which is as it were the treasury of life, it is made liquid, and is dispens'd through the body from thence, being fraught with spirits, as with balsm, and that all things do depend upon the motional pulsation of the heart.
>
> So the heart is the beginning of life, the Sun of the Microcosm, as for the sake of comparison the Sun deserves to be call'd the heart of the world, by whose vertue and pulsation, the blood is mov'd, perfected, made vegetable [*sc.* animated], and is defended from corruption and clotting; and this familiar household-god doth his duty to the whole body, by nourishing, cherishing, and vegetating [*sc.* animating], being the foundation of life and author of all (pp. 59–60).

The meaning which Harvey attaches to various of these expressions, such as 'natural heat . . . the treasury of life', blood 'fraught with spirits', 'made vegetable', will become clearer in what follows.

Similar ideas to these Harvey also propounds in *De motu cordis*, cap. 15. Innate heat distinguishes what is living from what is dead; innate heat must have a locus in the body from which warmth and life flow as from a source (*ab origine*) into all the parts, from which nourishment comes and on which depend concoction and nutrition and all living (*vegetatio*); the heart is this place and it is the principle (*principium*) of life. The heart gives motion and spirit to the blood. Motion is that which generates heat and spirits in all the parts. To recover heat and motion, the blood must return to the heart. So long as the heart remains without hurt (*illeso*), life and health can be recovered by the body.

There is, furthermore, the possiblity in this passage that Harvey is not only alluding but subscribing to the Aristotelian notion that the heart is 'sensitive', that is capable of sensation, and so the seat of the emotions or passions. I suggested above,[15] that he is thinking in more physical terms, but the alternative possibility should not be overlooked. It could equally well be true that because he considers the heart as 'senstitive' in 1628, he, therefore, suggests that all affections or passions of the rational soul (*animi pathema*[16]) which disturb the mind with sorrow, joy, hope or anxiety reach the heart and disturb its natural constitution with regard to its temperament (*temperies*) and its pulsation, and all else.[17]

One of the reasons for which the heart was thought to rank higher than the liver was that it was the only organ in the body in which blood was to be found not contained within vessels. Hence the notion that the heart acted as a storage cistern and kept the blood for the general use of the body, or, as was frequently said, for the common weal. Now every animal depends for its existence on nourishment which has been concocted and perfected in the body to be made suitable for use by the different parts and for their special needs. Various kinds of nourishment are necessary and are, therefore, concocted and perfected in different parts of the body; but all concoction depends upon heat. Different parts of the body use different heats, but the most perfect form of nourishment is produced where innate heat is most perfect and that is in the heart. Moreover, the heart is the only organ which can distribute this perfected nourishment to all the parts. (Its own supply is catered for by the coronary veins and arteries.) This idea also finds expression in *De motu cordis* (cap. 15, pp. 94–5), and Harvey follows it with the re-statement of his view that the heart acts as the propulsor of blood.

The next statement which Harvey makes on the use of the circulation adds nothing to what has already been said, but, as it is couched in the form of a question, it is permissible to regard it as indicating a certain doubt in his own mind as to its truth. It occurs in the passage added to the Anatomical Lectures, probably during the 1630s.

> And for this reason Δ it is certain that the perpetual movement of the blood in a circle is caused by the heart beat. Why? Is it for the sake of nutrition, or is it rather for the preservation of the blood and of the limbs by means of the infused heat? And the blood by turns heating the limbs and when it is made cold is warmed by the heart (p. 273).

As we have already seen, in 1636, Harvey was writing to Hofmann and side-stepping the issue of the purpose of the circulation with a plea that the phenomenon be first accepted before its purpose is discussed. And this he says again in the Second Letter to Riolan. In his letter to Hofmann, Harvey merely repeats what he had said in *De motu cordis* about the parts being warmed by means of the heat inflowing with the blood from the heart, and conversely, the blood suffering some detriment in the parts and returning to the heart, the 'fountain of heat', to regain its perfection. 'But whether this be so or not, I openly declare that I have not yet proved or even said much about.' By the time that he wrote the First Letter to Riolan, however, Harvey seems to have become convinced that this is in effect the chief use of the circulation. When feet and hands become cold like ice and blue, they can only be warmed by the circulation. The chilled blood which had lost its spirits and its heat is driven out

> and in its place, new, warm, and spiritous blood flowing in from the arteries doth foment and rewarm the parts and restore to them motion and sense [*sc.* sensation]; for they should never be renewed or restored by external heat, no more than the members of dead persons, unless some internal influent warmth did revivify them. This indeed is the chief use and end of the Circulation of the blood for whose sake the blood is driven in a circle and turned around in a continual course and perpetual inflowing; namely, that all the parts depending upon it might be by its prime innate heat preserved in life and in their own vital and vegetative essence and perform all their functions, whilst (as the Naturalists

say) they are sustained and actuated by influent heat and vital spirits; so by the grace of two extremities, heat and cold, the temperament [*sc.* temperature, *temperies*] of the bodies of creatures is kept in its mediocrity; for as the breathing in of air does temper the too much heat of the blood in the lungs, and in the centre of the body, and causes the eventilation [*sc.* dissipation] of suffocating fumes; so also the blood being hot, and cast out through the arteries into the whole body, does foment and nourish the extremities and sustain them in living creatures, and hinders them to be extinguish'd by the force of outward cold (pp. 134–5).

The chief use of the circulation of the blood then, in Harvey's opinion and other words, is to maintain the temperature of the body at a constant level.

Harvey devotes the whole of cap. 71 of his *De generatione* to the problem of innate heat. It may have been one of the latest chapters of this book to have been written. It certainly contains his fullest account of the subject and much that he there says is also to be found in his Second Letter to Riolan. In brief, it seems that during the course of his life he moved away from the complete acceptance of the Aristotelian notion that innate heat had its primary source in the heart, to the view that it is primarily present in the blood and consequently only had its seat in the heart by virtue of the blood which is there to be found. The problem is bound up with the question of the existence of spirits and with the idea of movement, or motive spirit. What Harvey has to say on spirits in this Second Letter to Riolan has already been discussed and it has been pointed out that for Harvey living blood denotes the existence within itself of heat and spirit, for without them it cannot be called living. That he had varied little in his views over the intervening thirty years is clear from what he says on this subject in the Anatomical Lectures:

But the philosopher holds rather (not as the vulgar do that spirits are distinct and separate from the humours and the parts as being engendered in different places or contained in different ones) but that spirit and blood are one thing, like whey and cream in milk, and following the definition of Aristotle the very word blood connotes the presence of heat as an accident in a substance which is essentially cold, just as does the word hot-water which implies as it were both steam and flame, the latter being the act by which the former is made actual [that is, to exist], and light is the result of something which gives light. As light is to the candle, so is the spirit to the blood and it has actuality in being made, like flames

223

from fire, existing in continual generation and flux. (The spirits are not from the external air.) (p. 293)

Elsewhere in the Lectures (p. 295) he writes 'spirit and blood is one thing'; and again, 'spirit, like flame, is in no wise separated from' blood (p. 319). In *De motu locali animalium* of 1627, he repeats the same view: 'Spirit is set in motion by the heart and flows through the arteries. Blood and spirit are one thing . . .' (p. 103). In the Introductory chapter to *De motu cordis*, he says it again: 'Blood and spirit make one body' (p. 6). His first remark, therefore, in this chapter of *De generatione* contains no novelty for it is merely to the effect that there is no need to look for spirits distinct from the blood. He then goes on to postulate that the blood is the first and only engendered heat. Blood is the first part to be made in the process of epigenesis, according to his observations, and as living blood betokens the existence of heat and spirit, this spirit is also at the beginning. Harvey now explains that by spirit here, he means that which conveys the power of movement. It is a notion which derives from Hippocrates according to whom all the parts of the body were to be divided into three categories, namely those which contain, which are contained, and which convey the force of movement. Blood is the first produced and chiefest of all the parts, and as it gives rise to all the others, it is possessed of all the powers of the others. There is no need to envisage the existence of any extraneous source of heat, for the blood can perform all the offices ascribed to the spirits and 'these spirits cannot separate from the blood even by a hair's breadth without their destruction' (p. 246). It therefore follows that the blood 'is both sufficient and suitable to be the immediate instrument of the soul (*animae*)' (p. 246). The innate heat contained in animals is not fire, but this innate heat present in the blood shares the nature of a more divine body, namely spirit. To explain the concept further, Harvey takes the example of three elements which perform the office of spirit, fire, air and water, 'and every one of these seems to be a participant in life or in some other body, by reason of their perpetual motion and flux, that is flame, wind and flood. Flame is the flux or motion of fire, wind of air, and flood of water' (p. 247). Because these three appear to have a kind of life, they can be said to act in a manner which is superior to the power of the simple element and so to share in a more divine nature. Now blood acts in a like manner not as a mere element, but 'in as much as it is possessed of plastic power [*sc.* capable of forming tissues, *virtutis plasticae*] and endowed with the gift of the vegetative soul, it is made the primigenial heat and the immediate and proper instrument of life' (p. 248). Blood outside the veins is a simple elementary fluid, but contained within the veins it is living and the immediate instrument and principal seat of the soul. It is the instrument of the Creator.

> Seeing therefore that blood acts above the powers of the elements and is endowed with such notable virtues and is also the instrument of the omnipotent Creator, no man can sufficiently extol its admirable and divine faculties. In it the soul first and principally resides, and that not the vegetative soul only, but the sensitive and motive also; it penetrates every part and is everywhere present; if it is taken away, the soul is immediately gone, so that the blood seems to differ nothing from the soul, or at least ought to be counted that substance whose act the soul is. For such is the soul, I say, that it is not altogether a body, nor yet wholly without a body; it comes partly from without, and is partly born at home; in some sort it is a part of the body, and in some sort the beginning and cause of all things which are contained in the body of an animal, that is, nutrition, sense and motion, and so consequently of life and death also, for whatsoever is nourished lives, and contrariwise. . . . And therefore it comes all to the same thing, whether we say that the soul and the blood, or the blood with the soul, or the soul with the blood, accomplishes all things in an animal (p. 250).

In *De motu locali animalium*, Harvey speaks of the motive spirit as that which distinguishes a living animal from one that is dead. He considers it to be the 'medium between soul and body' (p. 95), and he ascribes to it the beating of the heart and the pulsation of the life blood. So movement is one of the acts of blood. To sum up, it seems that for Harvey the word blood, when applied to the liquid which is in the veins and arteries of a living creature, denotes the presence of: one, internal, innate heat as a necessity for its existence and to provide it with the power to be an instrument of concoction; two, spirit, or motive spirit, which denotes its capacity to live and to be the instrument, in the Aristotelian sense, for the formation of other instruments, or in the embryological, for the formation of other tissues; three, soul, that is the capacity to give and foster life in all its aspects; the vegetative soul as found in the humblest plant, the animal soul as that which distinguishes an animal from a plant, and the rational soul as that which distinguishes a man from all other animals. Soul acts through the medium of spirit, but spirit cannot be separated from blood.

225

Harvey is therefore led to believe that because in his observations on the incubating egg he has seen that what he believes to be blood is the first part to move and therefore to live, the notions which in the Aristotelian way of thinking were attributed to the heart, should be reassigned to the blood. That he was already thinking along these lines as early as 1616 is evident from his statement in the Anatomical Lectures, after saying that blood is the author of the viscera, 'The soul is in the blood. Innate heat is the author of life and where it most abounds there it exists principally and primarily' (p. 127). And this identical view he repeats in *De generatione*, cap. 51: 'Life therefore exists in the blood (as we read in Holy Scripture), because in it life and soul do first dawn and last set' (p. 151). The reference to the Scriptures is to Leviticus xvii, verses 11 and 14: 'For the life of the flesh is the blood', and 'For it is the life of all flesh; the blood of it is the life thereof.' In both verses the Vulgate uses the word *anima*, which by the Jacobean translators was rendered 'life'. Harvey also uses the word *anima*, but it would seem to be erroneous to suggest that he was using it in any different sense from that of the author of Leviticus. There is no suggestion anywhere in his writings that he is thinking of the immortal soul of man in the Christian sense. Maybe he side-steps the issue deliberately; maybe as a biologist, with an intense desire to understand the mystery of life in a living animal, he deliberately separated his thinking on this from his thinking on religious and specifically Christian topics. Everything that he writes about the 'soul' has to do with the living animal. And when he says that when the blood dies the soul dies too, this does not mean that he is using the word 'soul' in the Christian sense, but merely in that of the author of Leviticus, the power of living in all its aspects ceases to be in the body.

Further, it is clear from cap. 57 of *De generatione* where he enlarges on his brief statement of 1616, quoted above, that what he is doing is making a premature and ineffective attempt to understand the great mystery of cellular and organ differentiation. He begins by saying that as we see the cicatricula enlarging in the egg and the colliquament being concocted and all things going on obviously with foresight towards the development of the embryo, there is nothing to prevent us from believing that innate heat and the 'vegetative' soul of the chick are in existence before the chick.

> For what can produce the effects and operations of life but that which is their efficient cause and principle [*principium*]? Namely, heat and the faculty of the vegetative soul (p. 189).

226

He then follows with another paradox to the effect that blood moves and consequently is imbued with vital spirits, before any of the organs for the formation of blood, that is the liver, or for movement, the limbs, are seen to exist. So also the foetus is endowed with sensation and movement before the formation of the brain, and it is nourished before the organs of digestion can be seen.

> Lastly, there is a mind, foresight and understanding not only in the vegetative part of the soul, but existing even before that soul, which immediately from the very beginning dispose, order and procure everything for the existence and perfect existence of the chick and with consummate art mould it to a form and likeness of its parents (p. 190).

It is not surprising that Harvey attributes the unexplained and inexplicable mysteries of generation to the power of the Creator. They 'surpass our powers of understanding not less than gods surpass men and are allowed by common consent to be so truly admirable that the dull edge of our apprehension can in no wise penetrate their ineffable lustre' (p. 82).

It now remains to decide whether in the end Harvey rejected the Aristotelian notion of the sovereignty of the heart in favour of a belief in that of the blood, or whether he effected a compromise. Both views can be supported by quotations from *De generatione*. The difficulty is to find reasons to support either decision.

Harvey's first explicit disagreement with Aristotle occurs in cap. 51, where he is discussing the primary genital particle. He first establishes the condition which the part has to fulfil to be considered as primogenate, that is, it must be the source whence vital spirit and innate heat, nourishment, growth, and life is given to the rest, where life first begins and last dies. The disagreement arises over which part fulfils these conditions.

> And therefore, as I conceive, being moved thereunto by a great many observations, the opinion of some physicians, whose philosophy is ill-founded, is to be rejected, for they hold that there are three principal and primogenate parts, namely the brain, the heart and the liver, and that they arise simultaneously out of three vesicles or bubbles; nor can I agree with Aristotle himself who concludes that the heart is the first genital and animate part. For the truth is, I am persuaded that this prerogative is due to the blood only, for it is the blood which is first seen in the process of generation. And that not only in the egg, but in every foetus and animal conception whatsoever . . . (p. 149).

Again, a little further on in the same chapter, Harvey repeats his disagreement with Aristotle:

> Being, therefore, even more certain from those things which I have observed in an egg and in the dissection of animals when they were alive, I conclude, against Aristotle, that the blood is the primary genital particle and that the heart is the instrument designed for its circulation. For the heart's business or function is the propulsion of blood, as plainly appears in all animals that have blood, and the office of the pulsating vesicle is the very same. . . . And hence the prerogative and antiquity of the blood appears, seeing that the pulse proceeds from it. . . . Nor is the blood to be called the primigenial and principal part only because in it and from it motion and pulsation have their beginning, but also because in it animal heat is first innate, vital spirit is first engendered and the soul itself abides (pp. 150, 151).

By the end of the chapter Harvey has proved to his own satisfaction that the blood fulfils all the necessary conditions to be considered as the primogenate particle. It is both the author and preserver of the body, and the heart is contrived solely for the purpose of ministering between the veins and arteries, of receiving the blood from the veins and propelling it into the arteries. It is the innate heat in the blood which cherishes and preserves the whole body.

> By all which it is most evident that the blood is the genital part, the fountain of life, the first born and the longest liver, the first seat of the soul, in which as from a fountain-head, heat first and chiefly abounds and flourishes, and from which all the other parts of the body derive their life and influent cherishing warmth. For that heat streaming with the blood flows through the whole body and cherishes and preserves it, as we have heretofor demonstrated in our little book on the movement of the blood (pp. 151–2).

In the next chapter, Harvey goes on to the question of the causes and use of the circulation, and expresses the hope that when he has finished, it will not seem as improbable and absurd as it did in Aristotle's time to view the blood as the familiar deity of the body, because in his opinion it is possessed both of sensation and motion, and these are the attributes of the soul. This attribution to the blood of the capacity for sensation, or of sensitivity, seems to be a crucial point in Harvey's thesis. Aristotle had denied that the blood was thus sensitive but had given this capacity to the heart. Observation could indeed show that the blood was insensitive; it did not feel anything as it spurted from a cut artery or vein. But to investigate the alleged sensitivity of the heart was a more difficult problem. Though Harvey could handle the beating heart of an animal in the course of a vivisection, he could not know whether or not his touch was felt. So it was not until he could touch the beating heart of the young Hugh Montgomery and learn that his touch was not felt, that he could know that the heart, like the blood, was insensitive. And it was this fact which seems to have made the greatest impression on him on that occasion.

> In the meantime, I will not be silent on this remarkable proof that the heart itself, that most principal member of all, appears to be without sensation (p. 156).
> Whereupon his most excellent Majesty agreed with me and acknowledged that the heart is deprived of the sense of feeling; for the young man perceived not that we touched him at all, but merely by seeing us, or by the sensation of the outward skin (p. 157).

It seems to me that this sudden revelation could have had some effect on Harvey's thinking. If the heart was in fact no more capable of sensation than the blood, then the one point in all Aristotle's conjectures concerning it which Harvey had so far been unable to control by his embryological observations and to contradict, could also be shown to be untrue. Consequently, the last thread which still bound him to some sort of acquiescence with Aristotle, no longer held. And by some gloriously irrational logicality, he could transfer all the supposed Aristotelian attributes of the heart to the blood. This then, would constitute his dethroning of the heart in favour of the blood. And the year in which this happened was about 1641, in any case before 1642, the year in which Hugh Montgomery succeeded to his father's title. (That being so, it is plain that to suggest that Harvey's change of opinion had anything to do with the politics of the period is to misinterpret the facts.) It remains, however, to be asked whether this is in fact what Harvey did; whether this change of opinion represents his final or merely his intermediate conclusion.

In the same chapter, he continues:

> Now if by the heart, Aristotle understands that particle which is first seen in the egg, that is to say the blood together with its receptacles, the pulsating vesicles and the veins, as one and the same organ, then I conceive he speaks most true. . . . But if he understand it otherwise, that which is seen in the egg will easily confute him, for the substance of the heart, being considered without the blood . . . is engendered long

after, and continues in the mean time white, without any infusion of blood, until the heart has been fashioned into the form of an organ by which the blood is distributed throughout the whole body (p. 159).

This is by no means the only occasion in *De generatione* in which Harvey seeks a compromise by interpreting Aristotle in this way. In cap. 46, when discussing the efficient cause of the generation of the chick and of the foetus, he refers to the ancient division of the parts by which some were considered genital or spermatic, that is to say present at the beginning, and others secondary, or formed, in that they arose later, and agrees that the heart has always been considered a genital part and refers to Aristotle's statement that from it the rest of the body is made, adding:

> and this is also borne out by our account. The heart, I say, or at least the rudiment of the heart, namely the vesicle and the punctum saliens, constructs the rest of the body as a future habitation for itself, and when it is built, enters in and hides within it, gives it life and rules it, and fortifies it with the superaddition of the ribs and sternum as with a bulwark. And it becomes as it were the tutelary deity, the first abode of the soul, the first receptacle of innate heat, the enduring focus of the animal's existence, the source and origin of all the faculties and the only solace in afflictions (pp. 126–7).

Again, in cap. 47:

> if the soul exists in the punctum saliens, building, nourishing and augmenting the rest of the body, as we have shown in our account, then it flows from the heart as from a fountain-head into the whole body (p. 131).

At the beginning of cap. 53 he again reiterates the compromise with Aristotle:

> if we admit the punctum saliens, together with the blood and veins, as one and the same instrument, visible in the first dawning of the foetus, to stand for the heart, . . . it is plain that the heart understood in this manner is truly, as Aristotle said, the principal and primary part of the body of an animal, yet its first and chief part is blood and that not only by nature, but in the order of generation (p. 163).

And he concludes the chapter with the words 'life is first derived from the heart' (p. 166). When, in cap. 55, he comes to discuss the order of the generation of the parts according to Aristotle, he points out that from what he has already said it is now plain that he has 'cheerfully embraced' (*nos ejus libenter amplexamur sententiam*) his opinion if, when

Aristotle says heart in this context, he means the punctum saliens and all the vessels full of blood (p. 175).

If it could be proved that caps 51 and 52 were written later than the others, then it would be possible to maintain that Harvey had changed his mind, that he had dethroned the heart in favour of the blood. But as he saw the young Montgomery before 1642, the suggestion does not seem altogether likely. Moreover, in the Second Letter to Riolan, a similar compromise with Aristotelian theory is also to be found. It occurs in the passage in which he is considering the rôle of the heart in the circulation, and criticising those who attribute everything to its power, not only the power of propelling the blood by its pulsation, but that of attracting and producing the blood and of generating vital spirits through its own innate heat, in short, those people who believe that movement, perfection, heat and every property of the blood and spirit are derived from the heart as being the first cause of pulsation and life.

> If I may speak plainly (*aperte si loquar*) I do not think that these things are as they are commonly believed; for there are many things which persuade me to that opinion, which I will take notice of in the generation of the parts of creatures, which are not fit here to be rehearsed. . . . Yet in the mean time I will say and propound it without demonstration (with the leave of most learned men and reverence to antiquity) that the heart, as it is the beginning of all things in the body, the spring, fountain, and first causer of life, is so to be taken, as being joyn'd together with the veins, and all the arteries, and the blood which is contained in them. Like as the brain (together with all its nerves, organs of sensation, and spinal marrow) is the adequate organ of the senses (as the phrase is). But if you understand by this word heart, the body of the heart, with the ventricles and ears, I do not think it to be the framer of the blood, neither does the blood have force, vertue, reason, motion or heat as the gift of the heart . . . (pp. 186–7).

It does not seem that Harvey is saying anything very different from his first recorded remarks in his Lectures where he concedes supremacy to the heart, not on its own account, but by reason of the blood which it contains (p. 249). Perhaps it is we who have not rightly understood the argument if we find any difference between this explicit compromise with Aristotle and the statement in *De motu cordis*, cap. 17:

> Nor must we disagree from Aristotle concerning the principality of the heart asking does it not receive motion and sensation from the brain?

231

blood from the liver? whether it be not the origin of the veins, of the blood, and the life? Seeing that those who endeavour to refute him omit the chief argument, or fail to understand it, to wit, That the heart is the first part to sustain life and contains within itself blood, life, sensation, movement before either the brain or the liver were made, or appear'd distinctly, or at least before they could perform any function. The heart with its own proper organs of movement already made, like as it were an internal animal exists from an earlier time. Once this was made, nature willed that by it afterwards should be made, nourished, preserved and perfected the whole animal to be as it were its own work and its dwelling-place; and that the heart, like a Prince in the Commonwealth, should be everywhere the ruler in whose person is the first and highest government; from which as from the source and foundation all power in the animal is derived and on which it does depend (pp. 114–15).

For all its glorification of the principality of the heart, this passage actually contains the expression of Harvey's compromise with Aristotle. 'The heart with its own proper organs of movement already made ... exists from an earlier time' seems to be a direct allusion to the punctum saliens, and the statement that is subsequently builds its own dwelling-house is directly reminiscent of the passage in *De generatione*, cap. 46, quoted above, where Harvey is explaining how this compromise is to be effected. That being so, it is difficult to maintain that Harvey's views on the relationship of heart and blood varied to any considerable extent throughout his life. There is, in his way of thinking, an antithesis between them. It is merely the emphaisis which shifts according as to whether he is thinking in terms of the circulation or of generation. But even when most concerned to stress the central rôle of the heart in the circulation, he does not forget that its principality is different from what Aristotle had supposed. It may reign supreme in the animal, by virtue of its office as the propulsor of blood, but its very existence depends upon this blood from which it was derived.

Harvey's observation of the movement of a heart while it was beating had shown him that the systole of the auricle coincided with the diastole of the ventricle, and that the systole of the ventricle in its turn coincided with the diastole of the artery. Once the blood was in movement because of the heart's action, this series of movements repeated itself for as long as life remained in the creature. The problem then was not that of the maintenance of the movement, but of its initiation. As systole invariably followed diastole, it could be supposed that in some sort diastole caused systole. It remained to decide what was the cause of diastole. For this Harvey's observations were inadequate; it was not a problem which his generation could solve for it lacked the necessary ancillary knowledge and the requisite technological assistance. Harvey does his best and resorts to his embryological evidence to try to find the explanation. At the very beginning of the embryo in the egg, he has seen the tiny white spot, which first blushes red and then begins to move. This he interprets as the existence first of blood and then of the punctum saliens. In this, of course, he is mistaken for the movement which he has observed is not due to the blood but to a thin layer of cells, totally imperceptible to him, which surround the blood. This observation, coupled with his belief that spirit is inseparable from living blood and that spirit denotes the presence both of heat and motive power, explains why on several occasions he refers to the 'obscure' movement in the blood itself, and why he attributes to this cause the diastole of the auricle and thus the initiation of the movement of the heart. His account will be found in the Second Letter to Riolan:

> The blood which is contain'd in the veins (as in its own hold) where it is most abundant, to wit in the vena cava, near to the basis of the heart and the right ear, growing hot by little and little by its own internal heat and made thin, it swells and rises like leaven, whence the ear being first dilated, and afterwards contracting it self by its pulsifick faculty, streightways drives it out into the right ventricle of the heart . . . (p. 180).

A fuller explanation of this view will be found in *De generatione*, cap. 51, where Harvey is considering blood as the primogenate particle. Having explained that the blood exists before it pulsates and that the pulse therefore derives from the blood, he divides pulsation into the two movements of dilatation and contraction. Of these he says that dilatation is prior and 'it is manifest that that action proceeds from the blood; but the contraction is made by the pulsating vesicle in the egg (as by the heart in a chicken), by its proper fibres as by an instrument destined to that use' (p. 150). The pulsating vesicle and the auricle of the heart are alike incited to contract by the blood distending them.

> I say that the diastole is made by the blood swelling as it were by the spirit contained within it. And so Aristotle's opinion concerning the pulsation of the heart (namely that it is made by a kind of ebullition), is in some sort true. For as in milk set upon the fire, and in our beer in which we see daily a fermentation, so is it in the pulse of the heart, in

233

> which the blood, as by a kind of fermentation working up, is distended and then falls down again. And that which befalls them *per accidens*, from an external agent (namely an adventitious heat), that is accomplished in the blood by its own internal heat or inate spirit . . . (p. 150).

If the blood is the first to live, it is also the last to die, and consequently, after the ventricle and the auricle have ceased to pulsate 'yet you shall perceive a kind of undulation and obscure trepidation, or palpitation, in the blood itself, the last evidence of life' (p. 151). As is to be expected, Harvey expresses these views also in *De motu cordis*. When the right auricle had ceased to pulsate and the heart was at the very point of death, 'there manifestly remained in the very blood which is in the right ear, an obscure motion, and a kind of spreading pulsation, for as long, that is to say, as it seemed possessed of heat and spirit' (cap. 4, p. 31). And in the same chapter he refers to the 'obscure beating' which is to be seen in the blood in the embryo before the formation of the heart and which persists 'after death' (p. 32).

With the merits or demerits of this explanation we are not really concerned. It was unfortunate that having denied Aristotle's views on ebullition in the heart, Harvey was compelled to accept some modified version of it to account for diastole. He is very careful not to let boiling actually occur for the emission of steam or air from the blood he knows is a falsity. What he probably saw was the fibrillar contraction of auricular muscle, with its referred effect on the blood. Moreover, his explanation does not account for the simultaneous contraction of both auricles, for the 'fermenting' of blood in the vena cava cannot account for the contraction of the left auricle. So in his brief account of the circulation in the Second Letter to Riolan he passes over this difficulty in silence with the simple statement that from the pulmonary vein 'the left ear keeping equal motion, time and order with the right ear, and performing its function, sends the same blood into the left ventricle'. He may have thought it a phenomenon similar to the simultaneous movement of the two eyes, and as inexplicable. One final strangeness about his account, is that it makes the heart depend not only for the initiation of its movement on the blood in the vena cava, but also for for the continuing of this movement. Yet he knew that an excised heart continued to beat in the absence of a blood supply, and it was with this very argument that Sir Kenelm Digby had shown Descartes to be mistaken in his views on the heart's action.

When Harvey said that there was no point in discussing the purpose of the circulation until its existence had been generally agreed, he spoke most truly. Neither he, nor any man in his time, could give a satisfactory answer to the question of its purpose, nor could he solve the problem of its initiation. His achievement was to establish the fact of its existence.

NOTES

1. The translations from *De generatione* are based on the English text of 1653 but corrected from the Latin. Spelling and punctuation are altered to conform with modern usage. The page references are given to the first, Latin, edition of 1651.
2. Keynes, *Life*, p. 330. Ent says the visit happened 'about Christmas last', and as it would appear that in the same Epistle Dedicatory, he alludes to the publication of the Letters to Riolan ('a small treatise of the Doctor's not long since set forth'), which were printed in 1649, the Christmas of 1648 seems implied.
3. C. Webster, 'Harvey's *De generatione*: Its origins and relevance to the theory of the circulation', *British Journal for the History of Science*, XI (1967), 262–74.
4. Keynes, *Life*, p. 344.
5. The text of Aubrey's Brief Life of Harvey is quoted in Keynes, *Life*, pp. 431–7.
6. Harvey uses the word 'uterus' to include the ovaries and Fallopian tubes.
7. It is tempting to think that this passage was written before the publication of Riolan's attacks, but Harvey may have thought that these did not greatly require an answer.
8. See above p. 107.
9. This was Hugh, the eldest son of the second Viscount Montgomery. He succeeded to the title in 1642, and in 1649 was commander-in-chief of the Royalist army in Ulster. He finally surrendered to Cromwell and was banished to Holland whence he returned to Ireland. At the Restoration, he was made Master of the Ordnance for life and was created Earl Mount Alexander. He died suddenly in 1663 at the age of 38. The episode which Harvey relates presumably occurred about 1641. It is recorded that Charles said to him, 'Sir, I wish I could perceive the thoughts of some of my nobilities' hearts as I have seen your heart'.
10. One other case is known in the literature before Harvey's time. Benevieni, in his *De abditis morborum causis* (p. 93) reports having seen a 'very small portion of the heart' when cutting into an old abscess.
11. The reason why Harvey chose hens' eggs for his experiments was because they 'are cheap and everywhere to be obtained, reasons that permitted us to make more accurate inquiry into the matter and allow others to have the opportunity to explore more readily and easily the truth of our statements' (p. 214). Both Aristotle and Fabricius used hens' eggs for their embryological observations and the practice

of examining hatching eggs daily to watch the progress of development is mentioned in the Hippocratic writings. On the other hand, 'there is more difficulty in the search into the generation of viviparous animals; we are almost entirely barred from the dissection of a human uterus; and to make any inquiry into the matter in horses, oxen, goats or other cattle cannot be without a great deal of pains and much expense. Those who are desirous to make trial whether we deliver truth or not, may test it in dogs, rabbits, cats and the like' (p. 214). In Ex. LVI Harvey refers to the number of dissections that he had made of the human uterus.

12. The fact that he could not find any trace of an embryo in the hind's uterus for two months after conception puzzled him greatly, and he described his findings to Sir Kenelm Digby who recorded them in his *Two Treatises* published in 1644 (p. 221). Harvey did not know that the peculiarity of deer is that they have a long, narrow placenta and a non-spherical embryo. This he did not see. Though it has sometimes been suggested that Harvey described the phenomenon now known as delayed implantation, this is not the case for it occurs only in roe deer and Harvey's investigations were certainly carried out on the red and the fallow deer. The only roe deer in the south of England at the date were in the carefully protected herds given to King Charles in 1633. See Keynes, *Life*, pp. 345–7.

13. See above p. 215.

14. *Lectures*, p. 273; the reference is to Aristotle, *De respiratione*, 479b 17–480a 15.

15. See above p. 143.

16. Harvey here uses the word *animus*, not the one with the Christian overtones *anima*. With the coming of Christianity, *animus* disappeared from the spoken language, and its place was taken by *anima* from which the modern French *âme* directly derives.

17. Harvey seems to be alluding to the nice balance of the 'humours' which had to be maintained if the body was to remain in health.

Appendix One

The Letters Exchanged Between Harvey and Hofmann, May 1636

M OST of the text of Hofmann's letter to Harvey, and many of its actual phrases are contained in CASPARI HOFMANNI Digressio in circulationem sanguinis, nuper in Anglia natam. Caput 48 Manuscripti Physiologici, printed in Johannes Riolan *Responsio ad duas exercitationes Anatomicas postremas G. Harvei etc. De circulatione sanguinis,* Paris 1652, pp. 357–64

Quae dicta sunt iam de motu sanguinis in arteriis, quia revocant mihi in mentem novum, et ab omnibus saeculis inauditum dogma quod Vuilhelmus Harveus, Medicus Londinensis anno 1628 sparsit scripta Exercitatione, ut vocat Anatomica, libuit hic obiter examinare illud. Vult probare Sanguinem ex Corde in arterias translatum et per easdem in habitum corporis deditum, assumi ex eodem in venas et remetiri in iis eandem viam usque ad Cor, ubi denuo coquatur, et per arterias in totum / corpus feratur, ubi iterum in venas recipiatur. Subrisi cum egerem, fateor, miratusque adeo sum, unam falsam hypothesin persuadere potuisse: tantum nefas. Huic cum respondisset biennio post Iacobus Primerosus, Londinensis, et ipse, qui in epistola praeliminari in os Harveo dicit, non maioris momenti esse quam vel Statica Sanctoris, vel lacteae venae Aselii, ὁμόψηφον me invenisse ratus contempsi negotium totum. Verum, quum postea intelligerem quosdam e Medicis nostris Scenicis (notatur Slegelius) applaudere Harveio, coepi relegere cum cura utrumque libellum, et in chartam coniicere quae Euripo isti recte obiici possunt. Haec nunc in publicum do, eo fine, ut adolescentes discant sugillare[a] portenta talia, et adhaerere uni veritati, cuius author et fundator est Deus, qui etiam diligit τοὺς φιλαλήθεις, et bonis multis cumulat, contra, qui mendacio, quod a Diabolo est, patrocinantur, semper miseri sunt.

Ut igitur quam ocyssime me absolvam, Hypothesis, cuius memini, est, plus Sanguinis mediante pulsu e corde in arterias pelli, quam vel restitui possit ab assumptis cibis, vel a partibus absumi. Pauca verba, sed ponderosa! Sed quomodo probabis, mi Harvee? Videris enim Naturam / accusare stultitie, quae tantopere erravit in opere pene

a. sugere

238

Caspar Hofmann to William Harvey

The things which have already been said about the movement of the blood in the arteries remind me of the new teaching, never heard of since the beginning of time, which William Harvey, a Physician of London, spread abroad in 1628 in an Anatomical, as he called it, Exercitation which he wrote, and so it has pleased me to examine this theory here in passing. He wants to prove that the blood is transferred from the heart into the arteries and through them is given into the whole of the body; that from the whole body it is received into the veins and travels back again in them along the same path up to the heart, where it may again be concocted and carried through the arteries into the whole body, where again it may be received into the veins. While I was reading this, I confess, I smiled, and I was much amazed that a false hypothesis had had power to convince, – such a wicked thing. When James Primerose from London replied to it two years ago, and said to Harvey's face, in the prefatory letter, that it was of no more moment than the Statica of Sanctorius or the lacteal veins of Aselli, thinking that I found myself in agreement, I condemned the whole business. But when I afterwards discovered that some of our matinée-idol physicians, notably Slegel, applauded Harvey, I began to re-read both his little books with great care, and to put down on paper the things that can be properly advanced against that tidal flood. These objections I am now publishing so that the young may learn to flout such monstrous fictions and cleave to the one truth whose author and founder is God, who loves those who love truth and fills them with many good things, whereas those who defend falsehood, which is of the devil, are always to be pitied.

To discharge myself, therefore, of this task as quickly as possible, the hypothesis, as I remember, is that more blood is driven from the heart into the arteries by means of the pulse than can either be replaced by the ingested food or absorbed by the parts. A few words, but weighty! But how will you prove it, my dear Harvey? For you would seem to accuse Nature of stupidity in that she went so far astray in a work of

primario, qualis est confectio et distributio alimenti, quo semel admisso, quid non sequetur confusionis in aliis operibus omnibus, praesertim in capite, sensibusque tam internis quam externis. Videris re ipsa damnare quod verbo laudas, ab omnibus acceptum Naturae elogium. Neque deficere illam in necessariis, neque vero abundare in superfluis. Videris Naturae dare personam artificis ignavissimi, et stolidissimi, qui opus a se factum et perfectum pessumdet, ut ne ocietur porro. Sanguinem enim omnibus numeris suis absolutum recrudescere, iterumque coquere[a] quid aliud est? Neque vero a recrudescentia abhorere potest, qui crambem recoctam tam studiose ornas, laudas, commendas. Sed auferamus τὸ videri. Siquidem ô Harvee Anatomiam exerces, non apud Senatorculos, Patriciolos, Foeneratores, Barbitonsores, imperitumque vulgus, quod hianti ore adstans miracula videre gestit: sed apud viros Anatomicos qui ipsi preceptores habuerunt ἀνατομικωτάτοις quo modo consulis honori tuo? Quid officii tui sit, nosti absque me, agere scilicet cum spectatoribus, more veteri, δεικτικῶς, hoc est, hoc videte; hoc ita sit, conside/rate; huius rei nec volam video, nec vestigium. Quin tu relicto habitu Anatomico logistae induis subito negas? Certe non uteris, aut uti iubes oculis, sed ratione et calculo, sollicitis computans articulis, quot libras Sanguinis, quot uncias, quot drachmas, necesse sit per semihorulae spatium ex Corde in arteriias transferri. Revera Harvee, persequeris πραγμα ἀνεξερεννητον, rem inexputabilem, inexplicabilem imperscrutabilem. Quod dico tanto maiori cum confidentia, quod fatearis ipse non semel quam difficile sit negotium et intricatum, systoles et diastoles Cordis, arteriarumque, ut possit certum definitumque quid statui a quoquam. Ratiocinari in infinitum licet unicuique: sensu (qui planissime hic requiritur) rationes comprobare tam facile non est. Et quorsum talia, ubi fundamentum nullum est? ubi, inquam, τὸ

a. coqui

almost prime importance, as is the making and distributing of food. And this being once admitted, what amount of confusion will not follow in all the other works she performs, particularly in the head and in the senses both external and internal. For that very reason, you would seem to condemn the universally accepted maxim concerning Nature, the which you praise with your own words, namely that she is neither deficient in those things which are necessary nor indeed redundant in those which are superfluous. You would seem to impose upon Nature the character of a most rude and idle artificer, who destroys the work she has done and perfected so that, forsooth, she should not be at a loss for something to do, for, to make raw again the blood that has been perfected by all her agents and then again to concoct it, what is it other than this? And it is not possible to disagree with this making raw again, you who so learnedly trick out, praise and commend this old tale. But here let us stop discussing this. If only, Harvey, you would not hold an anatomy in front of jacks-in-office, petty lordlings, money-lenders, barbers and such like ignorant rabble, who, standing around open-mouthed, blab that they have seen miracles, but in front of men who are anatomists and themselves had masters who were highly skilled in anatomy, ἀνατομικωτατοίς. How do you take care of your own reputation? You know without me what belongs to your office, that is to work with the spectators according to the ancient manner by direct demonstration, δεικτικῶς : this is, behold it; that it should be thus, consider. Of this phenomenon, I do not see the slightest trace. Why do you deny that you have doffed the habit of an anatomist and suddenly put on that of logistician? Of a truth, you do not use your eyes or command them to be used, but instead rely on reasoning and calculation, reckoning at carefully selected moments how many pounds of blood, how many ounces, how many drachms have to be transferred from the heart into the arteries in the space of one little half hour. Truly Harvey, you are pursuing a fact which cannot be investigated, a thing which is incalculable, inexplicable, unknowable. And I say this with all the more confidence since you yourself confess more than once how difficult and perplexing a matter it is to distinguish between the systole and diastole of the heart and of the arteries so that anything certain and incontrovertible can be established from any particular point. Any man may argue for ever, but it is not so easy to prove the arguments from observation, which is here most fully required. And for what purpose is all this for which there is no foundation? where,

241

ὅτι non constat, ubi in alto Naturae puteo absconditum est, ubi lucidiss-
ime rationes in contrarium sunt. Et quid (dicat aliquis) Primerosus
adhaec? Negat multum Sanguinis hic esse, imo disertè asserit parum
esse, sed videri multum ob intumescentiam, sive (ut ego loquerer)
ebullitionem. Amplexus logisticam adversarii ab unciis et drachmis
ad grana venit. / Fustra in aeternum.

Deceptio ut superiore capite dixi, inde est, quod uterque sibi imagin-
atur, Tamesin aliquem, in quo quemadmodum unda trudit undam que
semper labitur deorsum, usque dum perveniat ad mare in quod se exonerat,
ita putant in arteriis fieri. Eique rei exitum invenit quidem Harveus,
introducta fictitia illa Circulatione. At Primerosus nihil invenire potuit,
nisi si non opus habet, et consistant grana ipsius in eo, quod ex Thoma
à Veiga dixi. Ideo repetere oportet illud: motus hic comparari debet
non cum fluvio, in quo ipsa elementi gravitas facit lapsum deorsum,
sed cum mari aut stagno aliquo, in quo ventus ciet fluctus. In hoc ut
verisimile est, semper absorberi aliquid aquae in littore, licet nemo id
metiri possit; ita hîc semper absumitur aliquid, quantum scilicet Veiga
dicit, quod ipsum restitutione opus habet. Huc sine violentia trahi
potest, quod infra de chylo arterioso ex Hippocratis libro de Corde,
dicitur: τὸ σιτίον ἐν τῇ ἀρτηρίῃ ἐν ζάλῃ εἶναι. ἡ ζάλη autem tam
Cornario, quam Foesio fluctuatio est. Eadem ζάλη, mea opinione,
nihil aliud est, quam pulsus, quem vetustas tribuere solebat, non
arteriis, sed Sanguini in arteriis eunti, ut ex Aristotele dixi pronuper. Et
haec quidem de prima Harvei hypothesi.

Altera est, quemadmodum plus Sanguinis, quam partibus opus est,
in arteriis it, ita partes ipsae supra necessitatem habent; hic Primerosius
duo urget; Alterum, esse hoc contra Naturae providentiam, que per
attractricem non trahit plus, quam oportet: Alterum hac ratione fiet,
ut partes laborent perpetuis inflammationibus. His accensere licet ea
incommoda, quae ego supra. Iam has hypotheses excipit Thesis Harvei:
Hoc ipsum superfluum, tam in arteriis, quam in partibus nutriendis,

indeed, the phenomenon, το ὅτι (*lit.* 'the demonstration that'), is not agreed, where it is hidden in the deep well of Nature, where the clearest reasoning is against it. And what, someone may ask, says Primerose to all this? He denies that there is much blood, nay more, he clearly asserts that there is but little, but it appears much on account of its swelling up, or, as I would say, its ebullition. Taking up the logistic of his adversary, he comes from ounces and drachms to grains. Eternally to no purpose.

As I said in an earlier chapter, the deceitfulness in all this, is that each man can imagine for himself, some Thames or other in which in some manner one wave follows hard upon another which always flows downwards until it reaches the sea in which it empties itself, and in this same manner they think it happens in the arteries. And the solution of this matter one Harvey found by introducing his fictitious story of the circulation. But Primerose could find nothing, unless it be that there is no need for it, and his grains agree with what I have said from Thomas à Veiga. And so it must be repeated: this movement must not be compared with that in a river in which the very weight of the element makes it fall downwards, but with that in the sea or in some stagnant pool in which the wind sets the flow in motion. In this pool it is very likely that some of the water is always being absorbed into the bank, though no one could possibly measure the amount; and so something is being absorbed here all the time, that is, as Veiga says, as much as is required to be replaced. Without doing violence to the text, it is possible to take in support of this what Hippocrates says in his book De corde, a little further on, on the subject of chyle: The nutriment in the arteries is in flux (ἐν ζάλη). Now both Cornarius and Foesius translate ἡ ζάλη as 'fluctuation'. In my opinion, this same ζάλη is nothing other than pulsation which antiquity used to attribute not to the arteries, but to the blood passing through the arteries, as I said not long ago, quoting Aristotle. So much, therefore, for Harvey's first hypothesis.

His second is this: as more blood flows in the arteries than the parts need, therefore the parts themselves have a superfluity above their need. Against this Primerose urges two points. First, that this is contrary to the wisdom of Nature, who through the attractive faculty does not attract more than is needed. Second, by this reasoning it would happen that the parts would be afflicted with perpetual inflammation. And to these can be added the difficulties I pointed out above. Now Harvey's Thesis follows upon these two hypo-theses: this same superfluity of blood regreditur in venas, et per easdem in Cor, ubi iterum coquitur. Hic ego cupio discere ab Harveo per quas vias ex arteriis in venas eat? Per fines earum non dices, non enim se contingunt, imo in cutem desinunt, porosque constituunt, per quos excrementa tertiae coctionis eunt, et aliquando sudor. Fit, inquit, vel medietatè per porositates carnis, vel immediatè, per Anastomosin. Ut fatear stuporem meum, neutrum intelligo. Non mediatam illam viam, quia Sanguis, qui vasis suis excidit, et iam actu nutrit, non regreditur: sed nec regredi potest. Non immediatam hanc, quia in partibus nutriendis ipsis nunquam quisquam somniavit Anastomoses: sunt enim in maioribus vasis, licet Harveus non ob/scurè repudiet. Sed dentur viae quaedam caecae, et a tot retro seculis ignoratae, quas primus aperuerit hic Anglus. A qua facultate fit regressus iste? A Cordis, inquit homo. Cor ego scio, apud Galenum lib. 6 *De usu partium*, cap. 15, Trahere omnibus modis, sed eo usque extendere vim suam, ad partes, inquam, nutriendas: hoc verò novum est inauditumque. Nimirum modi illi trahendi pertinent ad Sanguinem, qui in se conficit: at ubi confecit, et a se ablegavit, imo, expulit mediante pulsu, quo ullo modo revocare potest? Maxime quia obluctatur vis partium tam attractrix quam retentrix. Nec est quod dicas, ablegari quidem per arterias, redire autem per venas. Illud enim vere fit, et est opus Naturae: hoc vero tuum commentum est, ô Harvee. Quin per venas non minus quam per arterias ablegatur. Quomodo igitur per easdem redire potest? Sed fiat, ad magnum tuum beneplacitum, ut quidam loquuntur, quo fine id fit? Ut iterum coquatur. Coquatur? Ergo-ne recrudescit? Nisi enim id fiat, quomodo non bilis potius generatur quam Sanguis? Nam Sanguinem ulteriori affatione facessere in bilem modo flavam, modo atram, est consensus omnium Medicorum. Sed sit ita, coquitne Natura / ut coquat? Et postquam secundo coxit? repetit tertio, quarto, et ita in infinitum? Quo fine? dico iterum. Hic enim est causa causarum, qua absente frustra dicitur, quidquid dicetur.

both in the arteries and in the parts to be nourished, goes back into the veins and through them into the heart, where it is again concocted. Here I would like to learn from Harvey by what paths it goes out of the arteries into the veins? I trust you will not say through their ends, for indeed they do not meet, nay, they end in the flesh and form pores through which go the excrements of the third concoction, and sometimes sweat. He says that it happens either indirectly through porosities in the flesh, or directly through an anastomosis. May I confess my bewilderment, I understand neither. Not through that indirect way [sc. through the porosities], because the blood which escapes from its vessels, and by this very act nourishes the part, does not return; nor can it return. Not through the direct way, because in the parts to be nourished nobody ever dreamt of the existence of anastomoses. But they do exist in the greater vessels, although Harvey denies it in plain words. But let it be granted that certain invisible passages exist, unknown to so many preceding centuries and first seen by this Englishman, by what faculty is the backward movement made? By that of the heart, the man replies. Now the heart I know, according to Galen, *De usu partium*, Bk VI, cap. 15, attracts by all possible means, but how far does its power extend? to the parts that have to be nourished? I ask you. This is indeed a new and unheard of thing. Doubtless, those means of attracting belong to the blood and it prepares them in itself. But when it has prepared them and separated them from itself, nay more, driven them out by means of the pulse, by what means at all can it recall them? Chiefly because the power of the parts opposes it, a power which is both attractive and retentive. Nor is it what you pretend that something is removed through the arteries and goes back through the veins. And yet this really does happen and it is the work of Nature: truly, Harvey, this is your false invention. Why is it taken away through the veins no less than through the arteries? How can it go back through the veins? But let it be so to your good pleasure, as some say, to what purpose is it done? To be concocted a second time. To be concocted? Does it not therefore become raw again? Unless this happens, how is it that bile is not created rather than blood? For all physicians are of the opinion that, in its final elaboration, blood is turned into bile, now yellow, now black. But let it be as you say, does not Nature concoct in order to concoct? And then afterwards concoct a second time? and repeat the process again a third time, and a fourth and so on for ever? To what purpose? I ask again. For this is the cause of all causes which not appearing, everything that can

Tu verò, ô generose quia ne attingis quidem hoc ulcus, sed silentio obvolvis, satius est ego quoque.

Conticeam tandem, factoque hic fine quiescam.

FINIS

H OFMANN'S letter to Harvey as contained in Richter, *Epistolae selectiores*, Nuremberg 1662, pp. 809-10.

Casp. Hofmannus, Guil. Harvejo.

Humanitas tua incredibilis, mi Harveje, facit ut non diligam te, sed deamem. Quo facilius a me impetrare potuisti, ut quod heri promisi, judicium meum de circulatione sanguinis tua, hodie praestem. Spes autem est, accepturum te eo animo, quo ego do, non ullo tincto livore, quo te pungam; nec ulla elato arrogantia, quo ultra te sapere videar: Sed simplici et candido. Quamobrem etiam spondeo tibi, si discussis nebulis, VERITATEM Hespero et Lucifero pulcriorem, ostenderis mihi, me cum Stesichoro, palinodiam publice canturum, et in partes has concessurum. Et ne ambages quaerere videar, sensum tuum puto esse talem, sanguinem ex corde in arterias translatum etc.

Heic ego tecum primum rhetorice agam: I. Videris Naturam accusare stultitiae, quae tantopere erravit, in opere paene primario, confectione et distributione alimenti! Quo semel admisso, quid non sequetur confusionis in aliis operibus, quae a sanguine dependent.

II. Videris re ipsa damnare, quod verbo laudas, receptum ab omnibus elogium Naturae; neque deficere illam in necessariis, neque vero abundare in superfluis, etc.

Haec ego volui, ut liberem fidem meam, quae accipies ea manu, qua ego dedi, Tu mi Harvee, bene age, et bene ambula cum Illustrissimo Comite Tuo, Domino meo Gratiosissimo, à chi baccio le mani humilmente.

Perscriptum Altdorfii 19 Maji MDC XXXVI.

be said is said in vain. But, noble sir, because you do not touch upon the delicate subject at all, but cloak it in silence, it is better that I do likewise.

Let me then at last be silent and having made this end here hold my peace.

THE END

Caspar Hofmann to William Harvey

Your incredible kindness, my dear Harvey, makes me now not only your friend but your debtor. And so you have more easily obtained from me today the fulfilment of the promise I made to you yesterday, to give you my opinion of your circulation of the blood. My hope is that you will receive it in the spirit in which I send it to you, that is, without any trace of ill-will with which I might vex you, nor with any high-flown arrogance whereby I might seem to know more than you, but simply and sincerely. For which reason I give you my solemn promise that if, having dispelled the clouds, you will show me the TRUTH more beautiful than the morning and the evening star, I will with Stesichorus, make public recantation and withdraw from the field. Now lest I be thought to seek an evasion, I take this to be your meaning: the blood is carried from the heart into the arteries etc.

Now here let me first try to persuade you with rhetorical argument. I. You would seem to accuse Nature of stupidity in that she went so far astray in a work of almost prime importance, the making and distribution of nutriment! And this being once admitted, what amount of confusion will not follow in all the other works which are dependent on the blood.

II. For that very reason you would seem to condemn the universally accepted maxim concerning Nature, the which you praise with your own words, namely that she is neither deficient in those things which are necessary nor indeed redundant in those which are superfluous etc.

These things I wanted to set down to discharge my promise and you will receive them from the hand by which I give them to you. Fare you well, my dear Harvey, and a good journey to you with your most illustrious Earl, my most gracious Lord, whose hands I humbly kiss.

Written at Altdorf, 19 May 1636.

The Latin text of Harvey's letter to Hofmann will be found in the *Journal of the History of Medicine*, xv (1960), 7–21.

WILLIAM HARVEY to Caspar Hofmann, the next day.

My most learned Hofmann, your opinion of me and of the movement and circulation of the blood, written so candidly, is most acceptable to me, and I rejoice at having seen and spoken with so learned a man whose affection I as gladly embrace as I cordially return it. In the first place, it pleased you to bring a charge against me in the terms of rhetorical argument and tacitly to reprimand me because it seemed to you that I falsely accuse Nature of an error of stupidity and impose upon her the character of a most rude and idle artificer in that she should allow the blood to grow raw afresh, and again and again return back to the heart in order to be concocted, and again and again flow into the whole body to become raw once more, and, to the end that Nature should have something to do, destroy the blood that has been made and perfected in vain. But truly now, truly, since I do not know where or when such things were either said or thought by me who have always thought myself to be an admirer of Nature's skill, wisdom and industry, it grieves me not a little to be taken for such a person by so fair-minded a man as yourself. In the little book I published, I merely assert that the movement of the blood from the heart through the arteries into the whole body, and likewise from the body through the veins back to the heart, is carried on continuously and without interruption, with such an outflowing and inflowing, with such quantity and abundance that it must of necessity move in some manner in a circle. But about concoction and about the causes of this movement and circulation, particularly about its final cause, I have never spoken but have omitted it altogether, deliberately, and this you will find expressly stated if it please you to read again caps. 8 and 9. Indeed, you proceed to complain that I am a

248

poor Anatomist and a poor Analytical Philosopher, simply because I try to investigate the phenomenon itself (τῷ ὅτι), without having established the wherefore (διότι). I will love you sincerely and most affectionately if you will read the summary of all my assertions in cap. 14. You will discover that I add to the phenomenon (τοῦ ὅτι) nothing but the general account of it, that I add to it no physiological speculation, that I add no causes over and above, nor speculate for what reason Nature should give this movement to the blood by means of the beating of the Heart. I do not deny that in cap. 8, I insert in passing for the sake of an illustration, as very likely may happen, that the parts may be warmed by means of the heat of the blood inflowing from the heart, and contrariwise that the blood may be weakened or suffer some accident in the parts, so that once again it returns to the heart and the fountain of heat for the sake of regaining its perfection. But whether this be so or not, I openly declare that I have not yet proved, nor even said much about. Likewise, in the last chapters, I infer from my anatomical observations and their consequences that a circulation probably occurs, but nowhere do I set out its causes (save for the heart moving with its own pulsatory power). You ask for direct demonstration, δεικτικῶς, and the testimony of your own eyes; it is plainly and truly written everywhere and I now declare to you that I have seen very clearly with my own eyes, and have very frequently demonstrated to the sight of the most perspicacious of very many of the most learned men by means of a dissection of human bodies many times repeated, the movement of the blood from the veins into the ventricles of the heart and from thence by the beating of the heart through the arteries into the rest of the body, and I have shown that then from all these parts the blood returns to the heart through the veins and that in such a quantity and with so violent a flow that there does not seem to be any grounds left for doubting the circulation. Do not take it amiss that I as an anatomist, and in fact a rational animal, need to use arguments derived from things perceptible to the senses and, what is more, selected from those which are admitted by all anatomists and to confirm the credibility of the account of the phenomenon as it can be singled out from an autopsy undertaken for the sake of this exercise for those who have never watched an anatomy with their own eyes or who shrink from such a sight. Does it displease you to know that Primerose is making calculations along the same lines as me, seeing that all anatomists acknowledge that systole and diastole, that is constriction and dilatation, occur in the heart, and that in dilatation the blood received from the vena cava fills the dilated heart, and in constriction of the heart occurs the pouring out of the blood into the arteries, these things they cannot deny being taught thereof by the texture of the heart, the structure of its valves and by many other things concerning it, and this process is a necessary one. If any transmission of blood, in any quantity at all, occurs at each pulsation, let them suppose any quantity they like (I make no reference to the amount I saw), and having calculated the number of pulsations, they must perforce concede that the blood goes round, immediately convinced thereof by the amount of blood they have postulated. But if you really have the inclination to see and experience for yourself, how much the single constrictions of the heart may send on, and to observe with your own eyes those things which could make your belief more certain, what happened in my case will appear as certainly, clearly and obviously, if the dissection is properly carried out, as you may remember you saw yesterday in Altdorf; and I have as great a certainty that the blood is diffused through the arteries into the whole body as I have that our Thames is poured out into the sea, and that the blood in the smaller veins goes into the larger ones and so on up to the base of the heart from every part of the whole body with as free a passage and confluence as your Pegnitz flows into the Regnitz or the Regnitz into the Main, as the Main and the Mosel flow into the bed of the Rhine.

Thus far the opinion of the best of men has passed judgement against me rather than against the circulation. Now, granted that I am a poor anatomist, the worst possible analytical philosopher, and that it seems to an upright and learned man that I have done wrong in what I have said of Nature. Therefore, the circulation of the blood does not exist! But this is a non-sequitur. You would deceive yourself, my very dear friend, were you to think me so conceitedly pertinacious on behalf of this or any other opinion that I could not bear words of contradiction without any trace of anger, particularly from my dear Hofmann whose face I had so longed to see that I could in no wise neglect the opportunity of visiting him, in whose friendship and discourse I was wont to take such delight and from whom to have this letter, written in his own hand, gives me such great joy. Indeed, there have not been lacking in England those who have striven in their anatomical demonstrations publicly to deny that I am the discoverer of the circulation, and quoting your writings, have rehearsed their belief that I was taught by you and by you instructed, so that I have had to make my defence by comparing our letters to each other with their dates in order to clear myself. Lastly, I accept with pleasure, gratefully and with thanks, what . . . namely, that the blood does not lie in the vessels like the water in your aqueducts, nor as our Thames in its bed rolls its waters straight to the ocean, but (a thing which is more correctly understood by the great Scaliger when he comments on the subject of flow in Aristotle, a subject which you foolishly say holds me captive) as any water in a pond or in the sea is always in flux; and just as the bank takes in moisture in no small amount by absorption, so do the parts which have to be nourished continually drink in the blood. Truly, my most learned and very dear friend, it would please me if you were now to smart for it. Surely, stagnant water does not flow? forgive me, I do not understand. Or as the water in the sea is in flux? The alternative proposition excites suspicion. But supposing it were as in the sea! There, there is such an inflowing and an outflowing at set times, and therefore the blood must go forwards and backwards in its vessels, and Nature would prefer the blood to be properly divided off and limited in the vessels rather than unlimited and disordered. Moreover, why do the lands of Egypt not take in as much moisture from the Nile as it flows past as they would if it formed a pool of stagnant water! I do not understand. Besides, how can the nourishment drawn out from the blood as it flows past adhere to the parts and be changed into cambium? it escapes me. The remainder of the points set out in your letter against the circulation are doubts of your own making because you refuse to accept porosities and invisible meanderings through the flesh. Without beating about the bush, you set up as obstacles to the contary movements of expulsion and retention, the manner of the transit and the ways and faculties which you yourself postulate, and you ask for the final cause and you say that you know that the resolving of doubts is the sign of a truth perfectly established. You say that the heart draws from the liver, why do the attractive and retentive faculties of the liver present no obstacle? and how does the blood come from the mesenteric veins to the vena cava, by what routes and vents, by means of an anastomosis, or in the very midst by means of the parenchyma of the liver? You never saw it, but you have no doubt that it may be. You do not hesitate to accept that the food is brought into the liver from the intestines through the tiny and hair-like ramifications of the portal vein, and that at one and the same time the blood is distributed into the intestines without any impediment, thereby affirming a contrariety of movement and a disorderliness. But I fear, were I to reply to each of your objections, this page would grow into a book and I would overmuch abuse your patience and so, heark ye, either you did not mark my book when you read it, or you have forgotten it, or else you did not understand me. If I remember aright, the objections which you have raised have their answers in the book, and they do not refute me. He who would grant the existence of the circulation either by means of actual dissection or by an argument from probability is not to be despised even though he may not know its ways or faculties, for such an investigation comes later, and from these considerations arise too much contradiction and elenchic argument. But since you ask for explanations to the end that I should free you, being convinced by them, from your doubts and not so that you should admit the phenomenon, ὅτι, itself, I promise to do so when you shall know the account correctly and agree to it, and to do it more strictly in accordance with analytical discipline. Now I fear that truly you deem me too little of an Analytical Philosopher, assigning as I am causes and resolving doubts for him who will not admit that the phenomenon may be; for this is indeed the sophistical method and, as it were, to speculate about non-being. But now my fingers ache with tiredness from holding the pen and other business calls me. I wanted to write these things to justify myself in the eyes of a very learned and much loved man and to free myself from the disgrace of so severe a criticism. And I assure you, most learned and very dear friend, that if you should want to see with your own eyes what I have affirmed about the circulation, I promise you this, which more becomes an anatomist, that whenever you shall wish it and the occasion serve, I will show it to you. But if you neither want this nor will be pleased to search into the matter by your own efforts in dissections, please do not, I beg you, disparage the work of others or ascribe it to error, or dishonour the word of an honest man who is not altogether unskilled nor a madman, in a matter which he has tested so many times over so many years.

Now fare you well, and see that you act with me as I with you, for I accept your letter in the sincere and friendly spirit in which you said you wrote it. Do you likewise to me who reply in a similar spirit. Nuremberg, 20 May 1636.

> Your
> William Harvey, Physician to the King and
> Professor of Anatomy at the College of
> Physicians of London, Englishman.

Appendix Two

Harvey and James Primerose

Harvey and James Primerose

WHILE this book was in the press, I chanced to read for the first time the letter addressed to Harvey by James Primerose in the introductory pages of his *Exercitationes et animadversiones in librum De motu cordis et circulatione sanguinis adversus Guilielmum Harveum*, published in London in March 1630. There Primerose says that when, very recently, he had been admitted to the College of Physicians and was attending the 'anatomical lectures on the diseases of the parts', he heard Harvey's discovery so praised by many people that they made it the equal of any discovery made in recent times, and, on the rumour that someone in Germany was going to refute it, 'an old man, speaking as it were from the seat of authority, gravely and proudly denied that there was anyone in Germany capable of doing so'.

Primerose was admitted a Licentiate of the College of Physicians on 10 December 1629, William Harvey himself being one of the examiners. On 11, 12 and 14 December, Helkiah Crooke gave the Goulstonian lectures on morbid anatomy. Primerose is certainly referring to this occasion. From what he says, it would seem that at some time during these three days there was a general discussion of Harvey's new theory and one would like to know who was the 'old man' in question. It is unlikely that it was Helkiah Crooke, firstly because at that date he was not old, and secondly because Primerose implies that this man was not the lecturer. There is in any case no reason to suppose that Crooke, who took no notice of Harvey's discovery in his own book, should have extolled it during the course of an anatomy. With regard to the 'old man', Primerose, speaking somewhat disrespectfully, expresses his amazement that he should think others incapable of doing what he himself could not do. So Primerose had himself taken up the challenge, 'persuaded and exhorted' thereto by the President. The President at this time was none other than Dr John Argent whom Harvey describes as his 'very dear friend' and who seems almost certainly to have been aware of the progress of Harvey's work from an early stage. Primerose's statement may not, of course, be entirely true, or perhaps Argent had a secret wish to see Primerose make a fool of himself. This he abundantly did in his book which is closely modelled on Harvey's, beginning as it does with an elaborate dedication to Charles I, followed by a letter to Argent as President of the College. The book, moreover, gives ample proof of the truth of Harvey's maxim that truth demonstrable to the senses and founded on observation cannot be refuted by ratiocination. Perhaps another independent witness of this scene will one day be found and the whole story become plain. Meantime, the interest of it, incomplete as it is, is that we know for certain that Harvey's new theory was publicly debated in the College of Physicians at least as early as December 1629.

Bibliography

HARVEY, WILLIAM, *Exercitatio anatomica de motu cordis et sanguinis in animalibus*, Frankfurt 1628. [Keynes 1(a)]

Exercitatio de Circulatione Sanguinis, Cambridge 1649. [Keynes 30]

The Anatomical Exercises of Dr. William Harvey, De motu cordis 1628: De circulatione Sanguinis 1649: The first English text of 1653, ed. Geoffrey Keynes, London n.d. (1928). [Keynes 25]

Exercitationes de Generatione Animalium, London 1651. [Keynes 34]

Anatomical Exercitations Concerning the Generation of Living Creatures, London 1653. [Keynes 43]

De motu locali animalium 1627, ed. and translated by Gweneth Whitteridge, Cambridge 1959.

The Anatomical Lectures of William Harvey: Prelectiones Anatomie Universalis; De Musculis, ed. and translated by Gweneth Whitteridge, Edinburgh 1964.

Text of Harvey's letters will be found in:

The Circulation of the Blood, translated by K. J. Franklin, Oxford 1958, also contains original Latin texts.

'William Harvey's Debate with Caspar Hofmann on the Circulation of the Blood. New Documentary Evidence', by E. V. Ferrario, F. N. L. Poynter and K. J. Franklin, *Journal of the History of Medicine*, XV (1960), 7–21, contains the Latin text of Harvey's letter to Hofmann.

Complete works:

Opera omnia, London 1766, 2 vols. [Keynes 47]

The Works of William Harvey, M.D., translated by Robert Willis, Sydenham Society, London 1847. [Keynes 48]

On Harvey:

H. P. Bayon, 'William Harvey, physician and biologist', *Annals of Science*, III (1938), 59–118, 435–56; IV (1939), 65–106, 329–89.

K. D. Keele, *William Harvey. The man, the physician, and the scientist.* London 1965.

Sir Geoffrey Keynes, *The Life of William Harvey*, Oxford 1966.
The Bibliography of William Harvey, *Cambridge 1928.*
The Portraiture of William Harvey, London 1949.

W. Pagel, *William Harvey's Biological Ideas*, Basel/New York 1967.

Harvey's predecessors and contemporaries:

Albertus, Salomon, *Tres Orationes*, Nuremberg 1585.

Arantius, Iulius Caesar, *De humano foetu libellus*, Basel 1579.
Anatomicae Observationes, Venice 1587.

Asellius, Gaspar, *De lactibus, sive lacteis venis*, Leyden 1640.

Bartholinus, Thomas, the Elder, *Epistolarum medicinalium a doctis vel ad doctos scriptarum centuria I (–IV)*, 4 vols, Hafniae 1663; Hagae Comitum 1740.

Bate, John, *The Mysteryes of Nature and Art: conteined in foure severall tretises*, London 1634.

Bauhinus, Caspar, *De corporis humani fabrica Libri IIII*, Basel 1590.
Theatrum anatomicum, Frankfurt 1605; 2nd ed. Frankfurt 1621.

Benedetti, Allessandro, *Anatomice, sive de Hystoria corporis humani, Libri quinque*, Argentorat 1528.

Benevieni, Antonio, *De abditis morborum causis*, 1507; ed. Charles Singer, Illinois 1954.

Bottallus, Leonardus, *Vena arteriarum nutrix a nullo antea notata*, Paris 1565.

Boyle, Robert, *A Disquisition about the Final Cause of Things*, London 1688.

Caesalpinus, Andreas, *Questionum peripateticarum libri quinque*, Florence 1571.
Κατοπτρον, *sive Speculum artis medicae Hippocraticum*, Rome 1601; Frankfurt 1605.

Casserius, Julius, *De vocis auditusque organis historia anatomica*, Ferrara 1601.

Caus, Salomon de, *Les raisons des forces mouvantes*, Paris 1615; Paris 1624.

Coiter, Volcher, *Externarum et internarum principalium humani corporis partium tabulae atque anatomicae exercitationes observationes que variae*, Nuremberg 1573.

Columbus, Realdus, *De re anatomica libri XV*, Venice 1559; Frankfurt 1593.

Conringius, Hermannus, *De sanguinis generatione et motu naturali*, Leyden and Amsterdam 1646.

Crooke, Helkaiah, ΜΙΚΡΟΚΟΣΜΟΓΡΑΦΙΑ, A Description of the Body of Man, London 1615: 2nd ed. London 1631.

Descartes, René, *Tractatus de homine*, Leyden 1664; Paris 1664.

Discours de la Méthode, Leyden 1637; Latin tr. Amsterdam 1644.

Description du corps humain, Paris 1648.

Oeuvres et Lettres, Bibliothéque de la Pléiade, Paris 1953.

On Descartes and Harvey, see Gilson, Etienne, *Etudes sur le rôle de la pensée mediévale dans la formation du système cartésien*, Paris 1930, pp. 51–101.

Digby, Sir Kenelm, *Two treatises, in the one of which, the nature of bodies, in the other, the nature of man's soule, is looked into in way of discovery of the immortality of reasonable soules*, Paris 1644.

Ent, George, *Apologia pro circulatione sanguinis*, London 1641; reprinted 1685.

Fabricius ab Aquapendente, Hieronymus, *De venarum ostiolis*, Padua 1603.

De formato foetu, Padua 1604.

De locutione et eius instrumentis, Venice 1601.

Tractatus de respiratione et euis instrumentis (Padua 1615); *De ventriculo, intestinis et gula* (Padua 1618); *De motu locali animalium secundum totum* (Padua 1618); *De musculi artificio et ossium dearticulationibus* (Vicenza 1614): a composite volume published in Padua in 1625.

Opera omnia anatomica et physiologica, Leipzig 1687.

The Embryological Treatises of Hieronymus Fabricius of Aquapendente, ed. Howard B. Adelmann, New York 1942.

Gale, Thomas, *Certaine workes of chirurgerie*, London 1563.

Galenus, Claudius, *Opera omnia*, 8 vols, Basel 1549.

Galilei, Galileo, *Opere*, Ed. nazionale, Florence 1890–1909, 20 vols.

Gassendus, Petrus, *De septo cordis pervio observatio*, 1635; Leyden 1641.

Guidi, Guido, *De anatomia corporis humani libri VII*, 1611.

Guinterius, Johannes, of Andernach, *De medicina veteri et nova*, Basel 1571.

Hofmann, Caspar, *De thorace*, Frankfurt 1627.

Apologia pro Galeno, Lyons 1668.

Digressio in circulationem sanguinis, nuper in Anglia natam, contained in Riolan, Jean, *Responsio ad duas exercitationes Anatomicas postremas G. Harvei etc. De circulatione sanguinis*, Paris 1652, pp. 357–64.

Laurentius, Andreas, *Historia anatomica humani corporis et singularum eius partium*, Frankfurt 1600.

Massa, Nicolaus, *Liber introductorius anatomiae sive dissectionis corporis humani*, Venice 1536.

Paré, Ambroise, *Anatomie universelle du corps humain*, Paris 1561.

The Workes of that famous Chirurgion Ambrose Parey, translated by Thomas Johnson, London 1634.

Parisanus, Emilius, *Nobilium exercitationum de subtilitate pars altera de cordis et sanguinis motu singularis certaminis. Ad G. Harveum*, Venice 1635.

Pecquet, Jean, *Experimenta nova anatomica quibus . . chyli receptaculum et . . . vasa lactea deteguntur. Ejusdem dissertatio anatomica de circulatione sanguinis et chyli motu*, Paris 1651.

Piccolomini, Archangelo, *Anatomicae praelectiones*, Rome 1586.

Plater, Felix, *De corporis humani structura*, Basel 1583.

Primerose, James, *Exercitationes et animadversiones in librum G. Harveii de motu cordis et circulatione sanguinis*, London 1630.

Academia Monspeliensis, Oxford 1631.

Read, Alexander, *The manuall of the anatomy or dissection of the body of man*, London 1634.

Riolan, Jean, the younger, *Anthropographia*, Paris 1618.

Anthropographia et Osteologia, Paris 1626.

Encheiridium anatomicum et pathologicum, Leyden 1649.

Opuscula anatomica nova, Paris 1649.

Tractatus de motu sanguinis etc. Paris 1652.

Ruini, Carlo, *Dell' anotomia et dell' infirmita del cavallo*, Bologna 1598.

Sanctorius, Sanctorius, *De statica medicina*, Venice 1614.

Servetus, Michael, *Christianismi restitutio*, Venice 1553.

Slegel, Paul Marquart, *De sanguinis motu commentatio*, Hamburg 1650.

Ulm, Franciscus, *De liene libellus*, Paris 1578.

Valverde da Hamusco, Juan, *De anima et corporis sanitate tuenda*, Paris 1552.

De la composicion del cuerpo humano, 1556; Italian translation Rome 1560.

Varolius, Constantius, *De resolutione corporis humani*, Frankfurt 1591.

Vesalius, Andreas, *De humani corporis fabrica libri septem*, Basel 1543; Basel 1555.

Opera omnia anatomica et chirurgica, ed. H. Boerhaave and B. S. Albini, Leyden 1725, 2 vols.

Andreas Vesalius' First Public Anatomy at Bologna 1540. An eyewitness report by Baldasar Heseler, ed. R. Eriksson, Uppsala and Stockholm, 1959.

Index

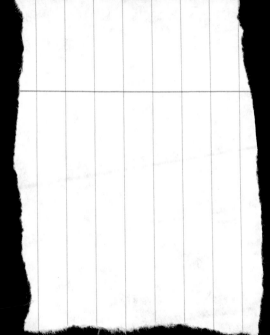